Psychiatry in Transition

Psychiatry in Transition
THE BRITISH AND ITALIAN EXPERIENCES

Edited by Shulamit Ramon
with Maria Grazia Giannichedda

PLUTO 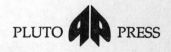 PRESS

First published 1988 by Pluto Press
11-21 Northdown Street, London N1 9BN

Distributed in the USA by Unwin Hyman Inc.
8 Winchester Place, Winchester
MA 01890, USA

Copyright © Shulamit Ramon 1988

Typesetting: Ransom Typesetting Services,
Woburn Sands, Bucks

Printed and bound in the United Kingdom by
Antony Rowe Ltd, Chippenham, Wiltshire

British Library Cataloguing in Publication Data

Ramon, Shulamit
  Psychiatry in transition.
  1. Mental health services—Europe
  I. Title
  362.2'094   RA790.7.E9

ISBN 0-7453-0177-0

Contents

'Deprofessionalized' Psychiatrists
Postscript: The Future

Acknowledgements

I would like to thank the working party which helped me in planning the book initially: Alec Jenner, Su Kingsley, Ron Lacey, and Tom McAusland. My thanks are due to the authors, most of whom wrote their contribution on time, but had to wait for so long to see it in print. In particular I would like to thank Franca Ongaro Basaglia for the generous permission to translate from the writings of Franco Basaglia.

Angela Bowering, who translated the chapters written in Italian into sensible English without losing much of the flavour of the original text, deserves special thanks. Ruth Carter typed the manuscript with care and efficiency.

Finally, thank you, Aelita and Teodor, for supporting me in the tribulations of editing this book through.

List of Contributors

BASAGLIA, Franca Ongaro, deputy at the Italian Senate.
BOURNE, Harold, consultant psychiatrist, the Connolly Unit, St Bernard's Hospital, London.
BRANGWYN, Gill, officer in charge, mental health, Greenwich social services, London.
CANOSA, Rocco, director in charge, mental health centre, San Paolo, Bari.
CECCHINI, Marco, psychologist, lecturer at the University of Rome and formerly director of the children's mental health service, Arezzo.
COGLIATI, Maria Grazia, psychiatrist, San Giovanni mental health centre, Trieste.
DAVIS, Ann, lecturer in social policy and social work, the University of Birmingham.
DEL GIUDICE, Giovanna, director, La Guardia mental health centre, Trieste.
DELL'ACQUA, Giuseppe, director, Barcola mental health centre, Trieste.
DE NICOLA, Pasquale, nurse, Cortona mental health service.
EVARISTO, Pasquale, psychiatrist, La Guardia mental health centre, Trieste.
GIACOBBI, Enrica, team leader, social work, Cortona health service.
GIANNICHEDDA, Maria Grazia, lecturer in law, the University of Sassari, research consultant to Censis, Rome.
HENNELLY, Rick, senior social worker, Tontine Road mental health project, Chesterfield.
HENRY, Paolo, psychologist, responsible for the health and social services in the area of the ex-psychiatric hospital of Grugliasco, Turin.
HOLLAND, Sue, psychologist, director of the White City Estate Mental Health Project, London.
JENNER, Alec, professor of psychiatry, the University of Sheffield.
KING, David, general manager, Exeter health district, Exeter.

KINGSLEY, Su, associate consultant, the King's Fund College, London.
LOSAVIO, Tommaso, director, Prima Valle mental health service, Rome.
MANGEN, Steen, lecturer in European social policy, the London School of Economics, formerly of the Social Psychiatry research unit, the Institute of Psychiatry, London.
MIND MANCHESTER GROUP
MEZZINA, Roberto, psychiatrist, Barcola mental health centre, Trieste.
PETRI, Silvana, psychologist, director in charge, the children's mental health service, Giugliano.
PILGRIM, David, clinical psychologist, head of counselling course, Roehampton Institute. President of the Psychology and Psychotherapy Association.
PINI, Maria Teresa, psychologist, Giugliano Family Advice Centre.
RAMON, Shulamit, lecturer in social work and convener of the social work course, the London School of Economics.
REALE, Mario, director, Via Gambini mental health centre, Trieste.
ROGIALLI, Sandra, psychologist, Arezzo mental health service.
ROTELLI, Franco, director, Trieste psychiatric service.
SALVI, Enrico, psychologist, Cortona mental health service.
SELIG, Naomi, psychologist, Napsbury hospital, Barnet.
TOWELL, David, Fellow in Health Policy and Development, the King's Fund College, London.

Abbreviations

b.m.	behaviour modification
CHC	Community Health Council
CIU	Crisis Intervention Unit
CMHC	Community Mental Health Centre
DHSS	Department of Health and Social Security
ECT	Electro-Shock Treatment
JPH	Judicial Psychiatric Hospital
MHAC	Mental Health Act Commision
MHC	Mental Health Centre
MHS	Mental Health Service
MIND	National Association for Mental Health
PCC	Psychiatric Community Care
PD	Psichiatria Democratica

Preface

Dramatic changes are now taking place in Britain and even more so in Italy, in the form and content of their psychiatric services. Recent media attention, the more vocal presence of direct and indirect users' organizations, and the greater interest in the psychiatric system by official authorities in Britain demonstrate that more people have become aware that what happens to our psychiatric services will affect all of us:

- as current or future consumers;
- as relatives and friends;
- as the nextdoor neighbour;
- as the councillor on a social services committee;
- as a member of a health authority;
- as local and national politicians;
- as workers in the field of psychiatry and related welfare services (home helps, health visitors, GPs, nurses, occupational therapists, psychiatrists, psychologists, social workers, members in voluntary associations).

In addition, more people are beginning to realize that psychiatry is not only a professional issue, but a political and moral one too, because it is about care for and control of a growing number of people who need our support.

On the whole, the book concentrates on people who suffer from severe mental distress, and services for them, and does not attempt to encompass the whole range of phenomena which come under the heading of mental distress. This focus is justified not only by the thrust of the current change in direction of policies about psychiatry which centres on this group: it is also the population which has been most segregated within our society.

For the first time the closure of our large psychiatric hospitals has become a real possibility, leaving us with two main alternatives:

- We can use it as an opportunity to create a new service and attempt to put right some of the wrongs of the old system.
- Or we can recreate the old system by establishing mini-hospitals and merely transfer the residents of the large hospital to yet another institution.

The slogan of psychiatric community care (PCC) has been in circulation since the 1950s, and is often used to cover up for lack of direction and resources.[1] It had been attractive to politicians from both the right and the left of the political spectrum, though the meanings given to it vary considerably. However, the slogan has been much less attractive – even terrifying – for those who may stand to lose by a major change in our psychiatric system, either in terms of power, employment or support in need.[2]

Both Britain and Italy are faced with the same central issues in regard to PCC, namely the processes and outcomes of de-hospitalization, de-institutionalization and normalization. These are long, cumbersome words, which do not mean much to most people. Yet we need to use them not only to capture the essence of the ongoing professional debate, but primarily to clarify their significance for ordinary people. De-hospitalization implies either the eventual closure of psychiatric hospitals or reducing considerably the very central place currently occupied by these hospitals in the British psychiatric system. De-institutionalization means that the new settings and structures of the psychiatric system are constructed in such a way as to prevent the continuation of personal and social marginalization of people who suffer from mental distress. Normalization is concerned with actively ensuring that these people will have opportunities for ordinary living.[3] As the text will demonstrate, while these issues are shared in the two countries, the solutions are diverse. Consequently, the stage where each society is in relation to the process of arriving at the main objectives of PCC differs too.

It is against this background that the comparison with the changes taking place in Italy becomes so important, for the Italians have opted for a far-reaching reform of their psychiatric services. Thus Italy has provided the Western world with a huge psychiatric experiment from which we can all learn, provided we do get the correct information.

For the first time, this text provides the British public with a systematic presentation of the insiders' perspective on the Italian reform. This contrasts with the often misleading and distorted presentation by some British writers previously. The contributions about

Britain adopt a critical, yet constructive, approach.

The objectives of this book are to describe the reality of the two psychiatric systems and to attempt to answer some of the questions highlighted by the description. The first part focuses on general issues related to the transition process and how these are reflected in the everyday reality of the psychiatric services and the public response to them. The second part concentrates specifically on the processes of changing the psychiatric system, including de-hospitalization, de-institutionalization and normalization, in relation to both users and workers.

The contributors come from different backgrounds and disciplines; from professional, voluntary, administrative and political activity. Some of them have experienced the psychiatric system at the receiving end. The diversity in background of the authors, as well as the cultural differences, has resulted in an impressive richness of ideas and information. They do not represent the majority of the group from which they come, as they are more likely to reflect the subgroup interested in changing psychiatry.

While not necessarily sharing the same views on mental distress or the psychiatric system, three common denominators are in evidence among the contributors to this volume:

• We all believe that mental distress does exist primarily as a personal experience of suffering and confusion within a specific social context. It is very much the outcome of the combination of the personal and the social. Likewise, each psychiatric system is the outcome of its social context and specific types of knowledge on mental distress. These two assumptions mean that even when there is a physiological reason for a specific mental distress, taking account only of that cause would be misleading and consequently harmful.

• Because we believe in the existence of mental distress, we also believe that society has to respond collectively to its members who suffer from it. Put in other words, we are not taking an 'anti-psychiatry' position, but a 'radical reformist' stance: we are calling for a profound restructuring of the psychiatric system as it is today, because it still tolerates the segregation and marginalization of so many people.

We are aware of the risks which may be incurred as a result of misapplication of PCC policies. Nevertheless we believe that de-institutionalization can be made to work with respect to clients and without harm either to them or their informal carers. We are also aware that psychiatry is a means of social control, but different psychiatric systems exercise different types of control: de-hospitalization, de-institutionalization and normalization are about using less control, and less of the coercive type. Unlike some academics of either Right or Left political convictions, we are not ready to sit on the fence in defence of our academic purity, pretend to be valueless, or wait for a total revolution, while change is taking place in psychiatry which affects people's fate.

• By emphasizing the social context in which mental distress exists and in which the psychiatric system is produced, we are also implying that the psychiatric system cannot be seen as a domain exclusively left to professionals. It is a sociopolitical system, as much as a professional setting, in which other social groups have – and should have – a say. For us, the most important among these other social groups are the users of the psychiatric services.

Let us say it categorically: we do not believe that any psychiatric innovation can be lifted from one society to another, because both mental distress and psychiatry are products of specific social contexts, which they in turn influence. Yet equally categorically we believe that knowledge and understanding of how another society has handled similar issues could – and should – be beneficial to our thinking about our own psychiatric system as a source of new possibilities and as one of the critical tests of old solutions.

Throughout the different chapters it has been attempted to provide a balance of conceptual, ethical and practical issues. The book contains many examples of the implementation of de-institutionalization and normalization work. However, while some of the examples are centred around an individual client, others are about the implementation of policies and collective work.

According to the biblical proverb one cannot be a prophet in one's own country; we therefore dedicate the book to Maxwell Jones and to Franco Basaglia, who – each in his own way – have dedicated themselves to changing psychiatry in our time.

References

1. Brown, P. (1985) *The Transfer of Care*, Routledge & Kegan Paul, London; Ramon, S. (1985) *Psychiatry in Britain: Meaning and Policy*, Croom Helm, London.
2. Lamb, R., Grant, R.W. (1982) 'The Mentally Ill in an Urban County Jail', *Archives of General Psychiatry*, 39: pp. 17–22.
3. For a further discussion of these concepts, see the contributions to this book by Giannichedda, Hennelly, Mangen and Rotelli. For an elaboration of the concept of normalization see: Brandon, A., Brandon, D. (1987) *Consumers as Colleagues*, MIND Publications, London.

Introduction

The Context of the British and Italian Psychiatric Systems

Britain and Italy had little by way of a common history up to the end of the Second World War. Although the countries were on opposing sides, the impact of the war was to become the turning point for the two social systems and their psychiatric components.

The following is an attempt to chart the main political, economic, and social developments in Britain and Italy from 1945 to the present day, the period in which the changes in the psychiatric system have been taking place.

Looking at the social context, 1968 is a dividing point between the immediate post-war period and the last two decades. Its significance will be obvious to Italians, but not for the British, for whom 1968 was merely an echo of what was happening in Europe and in the US. Nevertheless, the issues which were then brought to the fore in the rest of the Western world have since become important in Britain.

By now both countries have a similar population size (55 million and 50 million respectively), are governed by parliamentary democracies, are members of the EC, have the same (high) rate of unemployment and share the place at the end of the list of EC members' spending on health. Measured by economic growth, Italy has overtaken Britain in terms of its gross national product since 1986.[1]

Britain: 1945–68
At the end of the war Britain was poor, but victorious. With American aid and British work it set out to recover its economy, rather than to innovate it radically. The recovery was successful in terms of leading to what has been called the 'age of affluence' from the mid-1950s and to a real increase in the material standard of living for most people.[2]

The real political change, which brought the Labour Party to power in 1945, was the series of social reforms of basic welfare services. The 'welfare state' was motivated by several factors: the wish of both main political parties for greater equity; the vision of a Britain coming out of the war as a country 'fit for heroes'; and fear of Communism. The emphasis on the universality of some of the new services and on lack of payment at the point of service-delivery were the most profound innovations. The availability of these services meant that working class people could afford to use them, leading to the hope that poverty and its related public and personal ills would be eradicated in the near future.[3] While the National Health Service became one of the symbols of a universalism, social services remained separate and selective, with a consequent stigma.

The prevailing optimism and the wish to improve on the past were common to both political and public opinion. The post-war period was one of greater openness to new ideas, rebellious notions and departures from the past. In relation to psychiatry it meant the introduction of psychoanalysis as an alternative explanation of mental illness, competing for cultural hegemony with the accepted wisdom of mental distress as a disease. Young people and women emerged as two social groupings to be liberated and treated with greater respect. At the same time, they were also to become two new consumer groups, in an era of consumerism. However, users of public services were not considered as consumers, but rather as recipients of professional advice.

The belief in professionalism and expertise has gone from strength to strength, with a socially diminished role for lawyers and an increased one for doctors. This belief was shared throughout the political and social spectrum.

Britain 1968–88

The trends set up in the 1960s were continued in the early 1970s. The plea for 'white technology' and modernization remained primarily at the level of lip-service.

Both the health and the social services went through major administrative reorganizations. Community Health Councils (CHCs) were established in the attempt to represent community groups. The different sections of the social services were incorporated into the large personal social services departments, where priority over all other client groups was given to statutory work with children.[4] The call for change was related to the disappointment in the welfare system, with its impersonal service, bureaucraticized manner, difficulty in accessibility for the really needy, its stigmatizing effect and the fact that poverty was far from being eradicated. All this applied to the psychiatric system too.

Two significant social norms have been modified considerably, and are still in the process of change: the sacrosanct value attached to the two-parent model of the family, and the heterosexual orientation. This is reflected in the finding that a third of all British families have only one parent and that there is greater tolerance of those whose sexual orientation is different from that of the majority – at least until the arrival of AIDS.

The attack on the welfare state from the Right which developed in the late 1970s views it as a misuse of public money for private ills and holds that the very offer of a public service is a disincentive to the development of initiative, 'free will' and choice.[5]

This radical critique coincided with the growing number of welfare recipients due to the economic recession and the lack of innovation in the British economic policy up to 1979. From then on a new line has emerged, that of increasingly cutting the level of public expenditure, creating more and more unemployment and giving greater encouragement to the private investment and service sectors. While the rich have become richer, the poor and the salaried middle classes have become poorer in Britain, much more than in Italy in the same period.

Yet ideologically the New Right has so far been quite successful in challenging the assumed gospel of the past and moving the whole debate on the economy and welfare further to the right than at any point before 1979. So far the alternative from the Left does not amount to much more than a repetition of past policies. Furthermore, being put on the defensive, the Left has found itself defending all the past legacy of the public services, including its less satisfactory components.

The British welfare system has a long tradition of being a voluntary, non-profit public service. This sector, which has been expanding since 1979, has developed since in both traditional and non-traditional forms. The latter includes self-help and consciousness-raising groups. Paradoxically, this development meets the wishes of the New Right and the New Left for allowing consumers a greater say and minimalizing bureaucracy. So far the non-traditional voluntary activity has been limited mainly to the middle classes, with the notable exception of women in the mining communities during the one-year-long miners' strike. This type of activity has been the model for the most recent innovations in mental health (see Sue Holland's and Rick Hennelly's contributions below).

Several direct users' organizations have either come into being or become more prominent in the last two years. As Davis explains in

Chapter 1, these groups are demanding that the user's perspective of the psychiatric system is taken as seriously as those of the other main participants.

The private, profit-making, sector is surfacing as a factor which needs to be taken into account in the psychiatric system for the first time since the First World War. With the active support of the current British government, private accommodation for ex-residents of mental hospitals is a growth area, and some private psychiatric hospitals are being established too.

How long the present contraction of the welfare system will continue and in what form it will re-emerge remains to be seen. People with disabilities continue to be marginalized in Britain today, but less than in the past.

Although Britain is officially a member of the EC, remarkably little interest has been demonstrated by the British public in the rest of Europe up to now. Will that ever change, beyond tourism, football and foodies?

Italy: 1945–68

Italy was defeated and conquered by foreign powers by 1945. Famine, destruction and corruption coexisted with individual and collective initiative and courage. The war and its outcome made people question all that was until then accepted as gospel. This doubting included religion, the role of the Catholic Church outside religion, Fascism and Socialism. Furthermore, the relations between men and women, employers and employees, governed and rulers, and the role of the State were questioned. As a result, Italy became a more pluralistic society, in the sense that groups which did not share officially in political power managed to get real power nevertheless.

Although formally a centralized administrative system was established, the deep-seated regional allegiances have kept the country divided, with a weaker central government than in Britain. Since the end of the 1960s each region has had its own parliament and has to pass regional laws to ensure the implementation of national legislation.[6] The possibilities of regional variations in interpreting and implementing national laws are therefore innumerable. The responsibility for establishing and maintaining welfare services lies with the region, and with the local authorities.

This process of empowering groups is best exemplified by the power of the Italian Communist Party, which has never been in government up to now, despite the fact that it consistently commands a third of all votes. That party played a crucial role in leading Italy's major social reforms.

In the post-war period the Right too went out of its way to follow a populist line, perhaps out of fear of the Communists, and possibly also due to the pluralistic and regional nature of the Christian Democratic Party, Italy's largest party on the Centre-Right.

The main thrust during that period was not on change in the political system or on social reforms. Instead it was focused on the industrialization in the capitalist mould of the Italian economy, largely run on pre-capitalist lines up to then, with some elements of a corporatist state economy during the Fascist period.

With some American money, but primarily with a lot of Italian initiative and greed, Italy moved into its 'economic miracle', based on the cheap labour of migrants from the south in small and large industries in the north. As everyone in the industrial zone became richer, little attention was paid to the lack of industrial development in the south, its poor peasants, or the nationwide rising corruption.

Thus the 1945–68 period was one of massive migration, with real economic, demographic and social changes. Also, greater attention was paid to developments in the Western world, following the guilt and the shame concerning Fascism, and the Italian mixture of viewing Italy as inferior to some European countries and yet as superior to them too.

Consequently Italian intellectuals are more aware of the rest of the world than their British counterparts. Moreover, the professionals are seen – and see themselves – as part of the intellectual elite, rather than as skilled craftsmen. They would see as part of their duties to be informed of developments in their field outside Italy.

The economic and social developments, as well as developments in other European countries, have led to the emergence of three social groups as bearers of the demands for profound social reforms: the students' movement, the trade union movement, and the women's movement. The fourth group which developed on this background and joined in were those fighting against the marginalization of the mentally distressed.[7]

Since the 1960s the notion of the warm, all-embracing Italian family has largely become a myth. Yet compared to the highly individualized British way of life, Italians spend willingly more time in collective activities, including the family, and believe in the power of the collective.

Italy: 1968–88
The 1970s saw the fruits of the pressure brought to bear by those newly emerging groups and the political parties which joined them in terms of social reforms: the decade is full of such legislation as the divorce law,

the right of women to abortion, the admission of handicapped children to ordinary schools, the 1978 mental health law, the 1978 national health service legislation. While most of these reforms were initiated by forces outside central government, the latter took them on as its own, primarily out of fear of being left out of the credit for reforming and of being forced publicly to adopt them at a later stage. However, the government's deep-seated reluctance meant that often the struggle to implement a reform once it was legislated was much more disconcerting than the first battle for legislation. In addition, the government used a variety of tactics in order not to implement major reforms (for an example, see Franca Ongaro Basaglia's description of the psychiatric reform in the Postcript). All of these reforms came into existence in a country which, unlike Britain, does not have a tradition of a reliable civil service, or of universalized services (for a description of the structure of the health and social services see Introduction).

The formation of the Italian national health service (and the psychiatric reform, which is the focus of this book) stand out as the more unusual reform in comparison with European trends. While other European countries moved towards health insurance schemes, the Italian NHS was created to overcome the difficulties which have arisen due to the large number of insurance schemes, which counted on the government to bail them out of financial trouble.[8] It was also established to ensure a more unified and improved standard of health. It was aimed at offering a joint health and social service.

The 1970s were an exciting period, where new ideas were tried out, where previously marginalized groups were emerging in public, attempting to move out of that state. With this the cultural recognition of the socially acceptable changed too. This has not necessarily been wholehearted, but the boundaries between the acceptable and the unacceptable have nevertheless been challenged.

Although Italy – an oil-importing country, poor in natural resources – suffered from the oil crisis of the early 1970s and the economic depression which followed, it was not until the early 1980s that the sense of an economic depression dawned on the government and the public. For the time being this has suspended the reforms. This is best exemplified in the case of the national health service, starved of resources, badly managed centrally and locally, riddled with conflicts between administrators, professionals and pressure groups, leading to diminishing credence in the public service and diminishing investment in it by all of those who are involved. Being largely part of the health service, the psychiatric system suffers accordingly.

While the rate of unemployment is as high as in Britain, Italy's socioeconomic structure has been more able to absorb the unemployed into either the 'black economy' or into small, family-owned and run production units. Thus although unemployment benefits are virtually non-existent for able-bodied people, there is no real pressure to provide such benefits. On the other hand there is the recognition of the marginalization of the young unemployed, drifting into non-productive and often self-destructive activities. Yet in contrast to the 1970s, no mass organization of these groups has appeared, despite – or because of – a large number of university graduates among them. Many graduates in medicine and psychology remain unemployed for long periods, or work without pay.

A Right-of-Centre policy concerning the economy and the welfare system is being pursued, though more direct state intervention in the economy than in Britain is in evidence. The internal corruption of the secret services and the connections between the Mafia and apparently respectable commercial and judicial circles form the most formidable challenge which successive Italian governments have been forced to face.

Despite the improved state of the Italian economy since 1985, the current impasse concerning the social welfare needs of the Italian population is expressed in two ways: (1) not taking into account and doing very little about the social changes due to the economic recession (for example, people returning to the south after becoming unemployed in the north); (2) not providing the encouragement to implement fully the reforms initiated in the 1970s. It is on this background that the Italian developments in the field of psychiatry should be understood and evaluated.

Historical Background since the Second World War

Until the beginning of the Second World War the similarities between the two psychiatric systems outnumbered the differences, based on sharing the clinical-somatic approach to mental distress, very much anchored within medicine and the asylum. The physical conditions differed, because Britain was richer and offered a public psychiatric service much earlier than Italy. In that country, many hospitals were run by religious organizations, whereas in Britain there were only 36 private hospitals left by the 1930s.[9]

Yet there were striking similarities in the physical layout of the hospitals, including the large and well-cared-for gardens, the regimented living quarters, and the predominantly custodial atmosphere. Moreover, the interventions used were very similar;

namely insulin shock and later ECT (electro-convulsive treatment, discovered and developed by an Italian) and some rudimentary forms of occupational therapy.

Developments in Britain

During the war years and gathering momentum soon afterwards, the regime of the British hospitals did change, to include open wards, more occupational therapy possibilities and in a minority of cases a therapeutic community. Psychotropic drugs were introduced on a massive scale at the end of the 1950s[10] while ECT continued to be used. A fairly high rate of discharge took place from 1947 onwards, though it was combined with an equally high rate of readmissions and first admissions until the mid 1960s, when the number of first admissions started to diminish.[11] A similar pattern exists today in which the rate of first admissions continues to drop, while that of readmissions is still accelerating. In 1985 there were 76,000 in-patients inside the psychiatric hospitals of England and Wales, and 42,000 in-patients in mental handicap hospitals. The main difference between the 1950s and today is in the considerable reduction in the length of stay in the hospital – from an average of ten years in the 1950s to an average of several months by the 1980s.[12]

The regime inside the psychiatric hospital has not changed much in terms of the overall passivity required of the residents. Open wards offer a more liberal regime in terms of the ability to move outside the ward, but no greater resemblance to ordinary living. There are more rehabilitation wards, to which people are allocated when they are assessed as ready to be prepared for discharge, rather than for the preparation to be an integral part of being in hospital. Therapeutic communities were a British innovation in the 1940s[13] but 40 years later very few exist and they are perhaps even more isolated from having an impact on mainstream British psychiatry than when they were initiated. These communities encourage the continuation of ordinary resumption of responsibilities, the sharing of everyday tasks, side by side with an attempt to learn to live together with others and hopefully sort out some of the basic difficulties in personal interaction. They offer more group therapy and a democratized way of living. While most of the communities exist inside the hospital, some voluntary organizations maintain such communities outside the hospital too (for example, the Richmond Fellowship).

The sector which developed in particular since the war is that of out-patient clinics for adults and children. It is here, particularly in the work with children and their families, that the influence of psychological approaches to mental distress can be observed. Two main schools of thought and intervention methods dominate this field, namely psychoanalysis (psychoana) and behaviour modification (b.m.).[14] It will not be attempted to outline the main principles of these two frameworks here, but only to suggest that they have in common the assumption that the cause of mental distress is rooted primarily, if not always exclusively, in our past and current relationships to the social world, in the way we perceive ourselves to be vis-à-vis that world, which is often represented by 'significant others', such as parents, siblings, teachers.

Therefore the methods of resolving the essentially psychological problems that we are expressing via our psychiatric symptoms have to do with a reappraisal of the most important learning experiences/ relationships and by learning a new repertoire of self and others' perceptions and behaviours. The main differences lie in the differing assumptions on the role of the conscious (as in b.m.) vs. the unconscious (psychoana) components of our existence, the importance of the past (psychoana) vs. that of the present (b.m.) in terms of where to locate the reappraisal, the focus on behaviour as the primary location and tool for change (b.m.) vs. the focus on the subjective emotional experience (psychoana). Both approaches disregard the social context conceptually and to a lesser extent in practice too.

References to how the clinics operate are made in the section on the current structures of the two psychiatric systems. At this stage, it is important to note that they follow the clinical model in the way professionals relate to their clients, even when not employing a somatic approach.

The introduction of psychological approaches marked an important change in understanding mental distress and in relating to people who suffer from it. The milder forms of mental distress have been much more culturally accepted in Britain since the war. They are seen as an expression of psychological problems rather than as a physical illness by the public as well as by professionals. Often mild distress is perceived as symbolizing the existential difficulties of living in the modern world, shared by all of us.

However, between 1945 and 1980, society's view of severe mental distress has changed much less. For most British people it continued to be perceived as an expression of an underlying disease. Yet it was gradually accepted that most sufferers from severe mental distress can be contained without constraints for much of the time, provided they take their medication. Thus major tranquillizers – which dominate the prevailing mode of intervention – have a cultural value, in the sense of convincing the public that under the influence of the drugs people who demonstrated severe mental distress need not stay for long inside a walled institution.

The move to psychiatric community care is primarily about a shift in the social place of those who suffer from severe mental distress, the so-called 'psychotic', 'schizophrenic', or 'chronically ill'. An element of fear of potential violence as well as of the apparent lack of logic in the way such people behave conditions social and professional reactions.

The other main development in post-war Britain is the massive increase in the number and social status of professionals working in this field, primarily in the public sector. In part, this development has been made possible by the very existence of the NHS, its rapid expansion in the 1948–73 period, and the power given to its consultants. However, the main reason for this change lies in the cultural shift of accepting the psychological component in mental distress and in the university training all psychologists and many social workers go through. The increased social status of non-psychiatrists means that the traditional relationships of power and prestige in psychiatry are questioned and that in many settings new patterns of inter-professional relations develop in which the psychiatrist is no longer the unchallenged leader. This relatively new situation is still in a fluid state, where the inherent conflicts over power and preferred types of knowledge and techniques are surfacing more often than before.

Since the introduction of psychotropic drugs and b.m. in the 1960s, and family therapy in the 1970s, no new major forms of interventions have come to the fore. Yet psychotherapy in any form is rarely on offer inside the hospitals. ECT and psychosurgery too are still employed in British psychiatric hospitals. This is not to say that innovations do not exist, as several contributions to this book prove (see Chapters 3, 11, 17, 19, and 21). However, they have yet to make their mark in the mainstream of British psychiatry.

Instead, British psychiatry is renowned for its research investment and output, primarily in the traditional fields of psychiatry and following traditional research methods.

The only conceptual development in British psychiatry after the introduction of the psychological dimension was the anti-psychiatry movement in the mid 1960s.[15] As with psychoanalysis and b.m., this text cannot offer a proper exposition of what anti-psychiatry meant. Suffice it to say that it refuted the existence of mental distress as an illness and the value of the clinical-somatic approach for understanding and intervening with people who suffer from it. Rather, anti-psychiatry wanted initially to promote the view of mental distress as a family unit reaction, where the family is expressing difficulties not only in internal communication but also in its relationships to society. Therefore the preferred method of intervention was for the person identified as 'the patient' to move out of the family into communal living in a group which tolerated and allowed private space and regression.

Conceptually it meant doubting the positive value of family life and the relationships in a competitive and exploitative society. The severely mentally distressed person was seen as the only 'genuine' individual, suffering for his/her attempt to rebel against the hypocrisy in which we all live.

The uproar in the psychiatric and civil establishment which followed was considerable, with both R.D. Laing and D. Cooper being made to leave the NHS, having suffered criticism alternating between having their views totally ignored and personal defamation.

The anti-psychiatry approach managed to rattle the British psychiatric establishment, but it did not lead to a critical examination: on the contrary, the establishment closed ranks and psychiatrists and politicians adopted a defensive position. At the same time, in its heyday – the late 1960s and early 1970s – anti-psychiatry had the support of young people and social workers and was related to other new social movements.

Until the 1980s, psychiatric community care (PCC) was treated by most professionals in Britain as a highly pragmatic concept, in which the location of a psychiatric service outside the psychiatric hospital turned it into a 'community service' with a multi-disciplinary approach.[16]

British politicians were always for PCC, or so they said, while in practice very little was done by them about it until the 1980s.[17] The current situation is discussed in the Postscript.

Developments in Italy

As already mentioned, until the Second World War Italian psychiatry was similar in essence to the British system, through the European view of psychiatry as an inferior branch of medicine, the segregation of the mentally ill into large asylums, the departure from the 'moral approach' and the constant move towards strengthening the ties with general medicine. Italian hospitals were often even less clean and less comfortable than those in Britain, while the regime was much the same. Perhaps the only notable difference is that many Italian hospitals were not built far away from urban centres, but on the periphery. That meant that with urban development, hospitals became situated inside the city.

Until 1968 admission was possible only through compulsory orders. Most wards were locked, many people were in straitjackets or chained to their beds (see descriptions in Chapters 18 and 22).

In the period of reconstruction after the war, more new hospitals were built and more beds added to existing institutions. Italian psychiatrists started to renew or establish contacts with their colleagues in France, the UK and the US. Those openly dissatisfied with the system were greatly influenced by the therapeutic community concept or by psychoanalysis.[18]

In 1961 Professor Franco Basaglia, until then a member of the faculty of psychiatry in Padua, left to become the director of a psychiatric hospital in Gorizia, a small town near the border with Yugoslavia. He made it clear to those in charge that the objective of the first stage was the total openness of the hospital structure. To this end he negotiated an agreement which gave him the right to open the hospital in due time, to provide a personal allowance to each resident, and to work there as he chose. Professor Basaglia, together with a small group of psychiatrists, nurses, social workers and one sociologist, started by initiating daily staff–residents meetings, which often lasted the whole day. Gradually, after two years, most of the chronic, psychotic patients began actively to participate in the meetings, which discussed how the institution was to be run. This focus was already a major departure from the therapeutic community concept (which is more concerned with the relations among the members of the community and the staff) as well as with the outside world. *The Negated Institution* gives some verbatim reports of those meetings, plus reflections of the residents on what the process was like for them.[19] An apt metaphor is that of coming back to life, after being given up as dead in spirit, if not in body. The hospital wards were opened and left open from then on, during the day and the night. In-patients were accompanied to the town initially, and later emerged on their own, to taste ordinary life again. Simultaneously, residents were organized in small working groups which performed ordinary work inside the hospital, for which the minimum basic wage was paid. For the first time, local artists came in and helped to organize workshops, residents went for holidays with staff, to shop for personal belongings, and so on.

The major difficulties encountered at this stage were with the staff, not with the in-patients. Staff became divided between those who enthusiastically wanted the change to continue and those threatened by it. The ordinary local population was enticed and encouraged to come to the hospital, to the cultural festivities organized there for all.

By 1968, the Gorizia hospital had become identified by Italian young professionals, students of all disciplines, and volunteers from other countries as an example of an alternative, more liberated world.

The second stage was to move residents out of the hospital and the eventual closure of the institution, at which point the local administration recoiled, negotiations failed, and the most important members of the group resigned, explaining in an open letter to the residents their motives for doing so.[20]

This was in 1972, by which time similar attempts were initiated in Trieste, Arezzo, Parma, Ferrara, Naples and Turin. In contrast to Gorizia, Stage Two did happen in most of these places, in different forms. In Trieste the psychiatric hospital was closed in 1977, some of its wards were turned into flats, seven mental health centres with six to eight beds each were set up (see Chapters 4, 8 and 18), with a skeleton emergency psychiatric service in the general hospital (eight beds) but no psychiatric ward. In Arezzo too the psychiatric hospital was closed (in 1978) although about 200 residents live as 'guests' in the converted premises. The concept of 'guest' may seem strange, but it means that all civil rights have been restored to these long-term ex-patients who continue to live where they have been used to but as free people receiving support from the psychiatric services. In Arezzo there is a psychiatric ward with 15 beds in the general hospital in accordance with the 1978 legislation (see details in the section on the legal base, below). Ex-patients live in group homes, in old people's homes, in their own homes. Very few have in fact gone to live with their families, though in many cases contact with family members has been revamped in the process of opening the hospital. Local mental health services exist too: the one working with children is described in Chapter 12.

This description hardly gives the flavour of the considerable richness, improvisations and innovation of the different Italian experiences. They are typified also by the informality in relations between professionals and users and among the different disciplines, and by the lack of formal therapy sessions in most places – which is not to say that therapy does not take place. At the same time, there are areas where the psychiatric service has changed little from its pre-1978 form.

Psichiatria Democratica (PD) was created in 1976,[21] as a movement of professionals dedicated to a radical restructuring of psychiatry. Neither a professional association, a trade union nor a political party, it acted politically locally and nationally when necessary, professionally, and at the level of supporting other marginal groups. During the 1970s it was not a unique organization in Italy (see the activities of *Magistratura Democratica*). Its existence highlights one of the major differences between the British professionals and their

Italian colleagues, perhaps between British and Italian cultures: namely the attitude towards politics. Not only the members of PD but their opponents too have long accepted that psychiatry has a political dimension in so far as some of the major decisions concerning the structure and content of the psychiatric system are moral issues, and it is not – nor should it be – only up to the professionals to take those decisions. In addition, for PD, there was the recognition that in order for psychiatry to change nothing less than a process of sociocultural change was required. This process had to reach not only those directly involved in psychiatry as users, providers, relatives or friends, but also the general public and its representatives, i.e., the society which had previously expelled psychiatric patients and which was perhaps now ready to reconsider its view.

From the beginning, Italian psychiatric reform was not interested in de-hospitalization *per se*, but as a first stage on the road to de-institutionalization. Therefore it could not afford to neglect the political and cultural dimensions. Also, because the movement was a minority within the established professional circles, it could reach a larger audience only by moving the struggle outside them.

The interest in psychiatry generated in those years among the media and the general public is still in evidence today, even though it is often used to highlight the shortcomings of the reform.

The law legislating the national reform (see pp. 23–4 below) was passed due to the efforts of PD, several Left-of-Centre parties, and the support of progressive jurists. It was the culmination of nearly 20 years of small-scale experiments which proved their worth.

Conceptually the Italian reformers have come to use very different perspectives from those employed in British social psychiatry. They had the benefit of the experience of the Italian socialist movement, the partisans' movement during the war and they were also rebelling against a stifling academic tradition. On top of all of that, they were working during the two most dynamic decades of the post-war period. Equally their writings show a knowledge of French existentialism, British social psychiatry and later of anti-psychiatry too (see Chapter 24).[22]

Thus the main objective of the restructured psychiatric system has been that of integrating those defined as mentally ill into ordinary social living, rather than curing them of psychiatric disturbances or personality change. As for the end product, we will leave it for the reader to judge after reading this book.

PD was – and has remained – a minority among Italian professionals in psychiatry. The majority is neither for nor actually against the reform, remaining primarily indifferent, shifting allegiances according to local issues and opportunism. The main opposition to the reform comes from traditional psychiatrists and those privately practising psychoanalysis or b.m.

However, on the whole psychoanalysts and family therapists attempt to find ways by which they can influence or directly work in the public psychiatric service.

Culturally and professionally, psychiatrists dominate the Italian scene in comparison to other social welfare workers. As described in Chapter 22, nurses have only recently started to have a full training period, psychologists are a new group of only 15 years' standing, and social workers hardly have access to university training (and the status that comes with it).

Since 1978, the situation has changed substantially because of the issues raised by a nationwide reform in a country with a long tradition of regionalization, and where the cultural process discussed above was just beginning. All new admissions to psychiatric hospitals were terminated legally in 1980; all readmissions in 1981. In 1983 there were 42,000 psychiatric and mental handicap patients, 36,000 of whom were still in psychiatric hospitals, and the rest in the post-1978 units in general hospitals.[23]

The issues raised above and everyday reality of the psychiatric system as it is today are documented in the text.

Current Structures

The description presented in Table 0.1 on p. 16 and in the text below is bound to be schematic and does not take account of the considerable variations within each country. It therefore should be treated as an indicator of prevailing trends. It has not been attempted to illustrate at this stage the range of conceptual and intervention approaches to psychiatry, service users and workers. These can be discerned from the text itself.

In both countries the bulk of the psychiatric services form a part of the national health service. In Britain the personal social services are currently expanding their relatively small involvement into mental health. In Italy most social workers and psychologists in mental health work for the health service, either as part of a psychiatric team, or within a separate unit in a district.

Table 0.1 The Psychiatric Systems of Britain and Italy

	Britain	Italy
General Health Systems	A national health service from 1948.	A NHS from 1980, incorporating all previous insurance schemes.
Health Service Administrative Units	Regional and district health authorities; community health councils.	Regional, area and district authorities, no community health councils.
Funding	A central government-funded service; nominal sum for medicine; private sector paid by the public sector for some services. GPs remain in private practice, contracted to the NHS.	Funded by central government; ticket-paid-for medicine; area authority carries financial responsibility, not by speciality. Private sector is paid by the public sector, as in Britain, but can continue private practice too.
Selection of Management Committees	Management committee is appointed.	Management committee is elected by communes' councils; represents political balance of power.
Main Components of the Service	GPs. GPs refer to specialist and to hospital.	GPs. Paediatricians for children below 12. Referral by GP to specialist and self-referral.

	Britain	*Italy*
The Psychiatric System	Part of the NHS. In some instances the psychiatrist, or social worker, is attached to GP firms. Child guidance clinics. Out-patient clinics in hospitals. Hospitalization in general. Hospital (25% of all admissions). Hospitalization in psychiatric hospitals. Some community mental health centres (CMHCs). the centre's work. Community psychiatric nurses who offer a domiciliary service in most areas.	Part of the NHS. Multi-disciplinary teams at community mental health centres (CMHCs); centres are the backbone of the service. Drop-in, self and others' referral. Children service as a unit of a CMHC. 15-bedded wards in general hospitals for psychiatric admission. Some CMHCs have beds. Day care as part of Day hospitals. Home visiting by centre staff.
Residential, Non-Hospital, Care	Hostels, private accommodation, adult foster placement, group homes, therapeutic community in a minority of cases, individual flats.	Wards converted to hostels in ex-psychiatric hospitals, group homes, old people's homes, individual flats.
Social Services	A separate department, usually responsible for housing, some day centres, some CMHCs, some counselling, and social work attachment to multidisciplinary teams.	A unit within the health service, or in some cases social workers are members of the CMHC.

Referral

- Britain: via a GP or a social worker to a specialist psychiatrist: need for an appointment usually; very few drop-in facilities; some telephone consultations with non-professionals. Emergency referral for hospitalization in a psychiatric hospital: arranged by a GP plus a social worker, and/or a psychiatrist and a relative.
- Italy: via a GP to a mental health centre (CMHC), or self/relative referral; no need for appointment, centres act as drop-in services. Emergency: via general hospital to psychiatric unit in general hospital, or directly to a CMHC, handled only by doctors and nurses.

Out-Patient Services

- Britain: Most out-patient services are attached to hospitals. They offer an appointment to see a psychiatrist or at times a social worker/psychologist, for a specific objective and intervention, for example assessment, prescription, injection, or psychotherapy. Most appointments are on a one-to-one basis.
- Italy: As CMHCs are walk-in facilities, people can come when they wish or as arranged for a specific or non-specific objective; they are likely to meet not only their key worker but other workers and clients. The centres are often used as an informal day care facility. Home visits are frequently made by any staff member, without an additional payment. Assessment, drug prescription and psychotherapeutic meetings take place. The latter are usually much more lively than the equivalent British sessions and less formal.

Day Care Facilities

- Britain: Considerable variations in number per authority, type of clients encouraged to attend, activities on offer, formalities of participation, and user's say in what is offered and how a setting is run. On the whole those run by the NHS tend to be more formal and more like a mini-hospital than those run by social services.
- Italy: Few facilities are designated as day care settings, either due to lack of resources or to objection to segregation from ordinary networks and artificiality of activities. CMHCs tend to run ad hoc workshops, aimed at a specific collective project, often related to a neighbourhood event.

Rehabilitation

- Britain: Rehabilitation wards exist in the psychiatric hospitals, aimed at restoring everyday habits and at times as preparation for work experience. Some day care facilities are run as industrial workshops; pay is minimal and does not come instead of state financial support.

- Italy: Preferred, but often not available, are the work co-operatives, which require real work and offer ordinary pay, with ex-patients as co-operative members, at times with non-patients too. There are also some pre-vocational courses and apprenticeship schemes.

Psychiatric Hospitalization

- Britain: Many wards are open, but quite a number are closed and it is very easy to transfer a person from an open to a closed ward. Some wards are run as therapeutic communities. Major tranquillizers and ECT are the most prevalent methods of treatment. Psychosurgery is allowed; its rate depends primarily on the beliefs of each hospital's senior staff in the efficacy of this method.

  The physical conditions in a British psychiatric hospital are better than in a pre-1978 Italian hospital. Yet residents are hardly given any autonomy over everyday details of their living, let alone their psychiatric treatment. (The figures on hospitalization were presented on p. 8)

- Italy: A number of psychiatric hospitals have ceased to exist, with their previous residents either moving outside or using part of the site which has been converted into group homes or small communities. Sites have not been sold off, but are used also for schools, children's nurseries, local CMHCs, offices for co-operatives, etc.

  ECT instruments have been removed from nearly all existing hospitals; no psychosurgery is performed. Drugs are prescribed, though quantities vary, depending on the prescribing ethos of the local staff.

  When a region intends to apply the letter of the law rather than its spirit, there are decaying hospitals, a skeleton of community mental health teams, and no implementation of programmes for restructuring hospitals. (The figures on hospitalization were presented on p. 15.)

Community Mental Health Services

- Britain: Only 50 such services exist in the form of centres run by the NHS or/and social services.[24] Those run by social services are more focused on group activities and counselling for people already known to have been hospitalized. The NHS centres have multidisciplinary teams which work primarily as out-patient clinics, though more group work and family therapy are likely to be on offer than in an hospital-based clinic. A third type, the resource centre, is a rarity (see the description of one such innovative centre by Hennelly, in Chapter 19).

As described in the Postscript, mental health centres have become fashionable in the last two years, since the likelihood of some hospital closures has become a reality.

There are some crisis intervention teams and social work and psychiatry input in general practice which focus more on work with non-hospitalized populations and/or on preventing admission.

- Italy: CMHCs are the main agency of the psychiatric service. Some have beds too. They operate as a walk-in service. They may offer extensive home visiting, ad hoc groups, outings, cultural events, and carry the responsibility for sheltered housing. In principle, they would see their role as ensuring that all the user's needs are being met.

As with the implementation of Law 180 in regard to hospitalization, there are considerable variations in the way mental health centres operate and the type of service they would provide.

Housing

- Britain: There are no provisions for people in a mental distress crisis who have not been hospitalized. Those discharged after hospitalization are legally entitled to local authority housing if, for a variety of reasons, they cannot return to their previous home. Hostels, adult foster placements and group homes are often used. Less frequent are individual flats or placement in a therapeutic community run by a voluntary agency, such as the Richmond Fellowship. With the government's push towards the privatization of the health and social services, many ex-patients end up in private accommodation. Most of this accommodation is unsupervised, unlike adult foster placements which, although private, are closely supervised.
- Italy: There are very few facilities for a pre-hospitalization refuge. Those that exist are offered by mental health centres with beds and in day centres (such as the one described in Chapter 20).

Most ex-patients who left the hospitals due to closure live in small group homes. Some of the elderly among them live in small old people's homes. There is a considerable housing shortage in Italy, which makes the task of finding housing solutions for people who suffer from mental distress daunting. As mentioned above, mental health centres are responsible for the various housing solutions.

Private Psychiatric Services

- Britain: Private consultation and psychotherapy are easily available but depend on ability to pay. There are very few private hospitals, but the number is currently growing with the encouragement of the present government. Private accommodation for ex-patients is an expanding area, funded as it is by the public sector.

- Italy: Private out-patient consultation and psychotherapy tend to exist mainly in large cities. There are private hospitals and clinics, most of which are for poor people. These establishments are usually run by religious organizations. Often they provide poor physical conditions as well as psychiatric intervention. Not surprisingly more of these exist in the south. There is no evidence to prove a growth of these institutions or of private accommodation in the post-1978 period.[25] As in Britain, the private clinics and hospitals, as well as private accommodation, are largely financed by the public sector.

Cost

- Britain: The British NHS is spending about £2 billion per year on its psychiatric services, of which £1.5 bn go to the hospital sector, and only £0.5 bn to services outside the hospital. The personal social services spend about 2 per cent of their annual budget on mental distress/health.[26]
- Italy: In 1982 Italy spent 1,245 bn Italian lire on psychiatry (one English £ sterling is equivalent to about 2,000 lire today). Only 82,000 million lire of this sum were spent on community services. However, as a large proportion of the current services on offer on the sites of the psychiatric services are those provided for the 'guests' category, the real amount spent on psychiatric community care is considerably higher than this sum would suggest. The private hospitals take as much as 391,000 million lire from the Ministry of Health.[27] Despite the lack of sufficient accuracy in the costing calculation, there is little doubt that the Italian service is financially less resourced than the British system.

Some research evidence suggests that areas which have developed their community service more, and either do not have a hospital sector or have a small hospital base, are spending less money per capita than those with a larger hospital sector.[28]

The Legal Base

Britain

Britain's latest mental health law, the amendments to the 1959 Mental Health Act, was passed in 1983.[29] Most of it consists of regulations concerning compulsory admissions. Following the 1959 legislation, but more firmly so, social workers play a major role in assessing people for

compulsory admission. In principle they have to satisfy themselves
that there is no alternative but for the person to be thus admitted. The
final say in every case lies with psychiatrists, as the social worker's
recommendations can be overruled by two psychiatric opinions.

The law includes mental illness, psychopathy and mental handicap as
categories for compulsory admission. It does not define mental illness,
leaving it to be done by professionals on an ad hoc basis.

There are two main innovations in the 1983 law: first a Mental Health
Commission whose function is to inspect physical conditions and legal
procedures pertaining to those under compulsory order was established.
The Commission was created in 1984, consisting of 90 members, who
represent the different professions involved, the voluntary sector and
community health councils. They are all appointed by the Minister of
Health. It was not seen fit to include representatives of service users.
Second the Commission also has the duty to recommend to the Minister
that interventions judged as likely to lead to irreversible damage to
patients will be put on a special list. Being put on the list implies a
requirement not only for the patient's consent to treatment, but also for
one independent psychiatric opinion, apart from that of the patient's
direct doctor. However, the psychiatrist can overrule the patient's
decision. So far only two treatments have been put on the list,
psychosurgery and hormonal treatment. The Commission is accountable
to the Minister but not to Parliament.

Research on how the Act has been implemented demonstrates several
problem areas, which include the use of section 136, guardianship, the
work of tribunals, and the special list referred to above. In particular,
the involvement of the police and social workers in using section 136,
which enables the detention of a person in a police station for up to 72
hours on psychiatric grounds, has raised concern about the
disproportionate number of young black men who find themselves in
custody and later in hospital through the use of this section.[30]

Recently, the Royal College of Psychiatrists and the Schizophrenia
Fellowship (a relatives' organization) have proposed the legislation of
compulsory medical treatment order in the community, which is
discussed in the Postscript. Briefly, the suggested order would be
enforced with hospitalization if people served with it would not
comply and refused to take medication. If such an order were to pass, it
would imply a radical departure from the present thinking about
hospital admission, which is concerned with treatment and the
prevention of risk, and not with the use of hospitalization as a means for
preventing the recurrence of a mental breakdown.

Complaints about procedure and conditions can be put to the

Commission and to the Mental Health Review Tribunals, which have existed since 1960. Tribunals' panels consist of a lawyer, a psychiatrist and a lay person. Hearings follow the procedures of most other tribunals (for example, people are allowed to be legally represented) but it is up to the panel to decide whether the person/patient lodging the complaint is permitted to see his/her own file.

The data available on tribunals since 1960 shows a low uptake by patients, a very low rate of cases where the request by patients was upheld as against a very high rate in which the psychiatrists' view was upheld by the tribunal (12 per cent vs 88 per cent, see Gostin).[31]

According to the law, local authorities have to provide aftercare services, including accommodation, on a permissive basis. This basis implies that each local authority can choose how much to invest in these services as against others. Authorities cannot be sued for lack of services, in the way possible if, for example, a school place is not available for every child aged 5–16 years in a given authority.

The British law pertains also to the four special hospitals with their 2,500 residents. But it excludes the 95 per cent of in-patients who are in hospitals on a voluntary basis or the many more who use the psychiatric services without hospitalization (currently estimated to be around two million per year).[32] The law does not set out guidelines for the structure and/or the content of the psychiatric services. Likewise, terms such as 'psychiatric community care' or 'normalization' do not appear in British mental health legislation.

Italy

Italy's latest mental health law was passed in 1978, Law no. 180/1978, officially entitled 'Voluntary and Compulsory Health Assessment and Treatment' and usually referred to as the law on reforming psychiatric assistance, or simply as Law 180.[33] The law states that:

- New psychiatric admissions to psychiatric hospitals will cease after 31 December 1979. No readmissions will be possible after 31 December 1980.
- No further building of existing hospitals, or new ones, would be permitted in the psychiatric sector from the date the law was put into practice (1 May 1978).
- 15 designated psychiatric beds per 200,000 inhabitants can be established within general hospitals, or in the CMHC.
- Community mental health centres need to be established by the regions throughout the country.

- People can be admitted to the new psychiatric facility (named 'unit for diagnosis and cure') or to a CMHC by a compulsory order for reason of refusal to be treated otherwise when treatment was deemed as necessary for the well-being of the patient, but not for dangerousness. In such a case the order has to be proposed by a psychiatrist, agreed by the local mayor and signed by the tutelary judge, for the duration of no more than seven days. The order can be renewed if convincing reasons are given in writing.

The law does not cover the six Italian psychiatric prisons with their 1,650 inmates (Chapter 14 focuses on these settings).

The responsibility for enforcing the law lies with the Italian regions. As already mentioned, the regions have a relatively high level of autonomy from central government. Each region had to pass its mental health law in order to implement the national Law 180. The striking unevenness of the degree of implementation of the law is directly related to the role played by each region (for details on the distribution of services in four Italian regions by 1984 see Censis).[34]

Article 7 of Law 180 requires the redeployment of all mental health workers. Workers were encouraged to move to work outside the hospital or to take early retirement.

Although not forming part of the written law, regulations were made as to the flexible transfer of monies within the system: money saved by the closure of a ward was directly used for opening/sustaining a facility outside the hospital and was not put back into the hospital's budget.

Still part of the non-legislated, but closely-followed, code was the abolition of ECT by the physical removal of the apparatus from all public psychiatric services. Less closely observed, but in evidence in mental health centres with beds and in small general hospitals, is the fact that even patients under compulsory order are kept in open facilities. Living with compulsory treatment in an open environment invariably leads to new rules and behaviour in both staff and clients (see examples in Chapters 4 and 18).

It is clear that the legislative basis differs considerably in the two countries. While the British law is typical of most Western legislation since the 1950s, the Italian Act is still an exception in legislating the structure of a new psychiatric system.

Given this exceptionality and the unevenness of the application of the reform throughout Italy it is not surprising that there are attempts to modify Law 180 (for a summary of the modification proposals see Cravedi).[35] The main change proposed is to establish small residential units (with up to 20 people) for 'chronic' patients. This suggestion is seen as an attempt to reintroduce long-term institutionalization for this group by those who oppose any modification. No-one in present-day Italy is calling for the reopening of psychiatric hospitals. Culturally the mental hospital concept has ceased to be a viable option.

While the debate continues with its ups and downs, it has so far demonstrated clearly that both the support and the opposition for the reform cross the boundaries of all political parties. Protagonists and opponents of Law 180 are to be found in all parties. The claim made in Britain that only the Italian Communist Party supports the law is incorrect and is used as a means to prevent a real debate on and a real change in Britain's psychiatric system.[36]

References

1. See *The Times*, 17 November 1987, supplement on Italy.
2. Bogdanor, V., Skidelsky, R. (ed) (1970) *The Age of Affluence 1951–1964*, Macmillan, London.
3. Titmus, R. M. (1958) *Essays on the Welfare State*, Allen & Unwin, London.
4. Hall, P. (1972) *Reforming the Welfare*, Heinemann, London.
5. Bosanquet, N. (1985) *The New Right*, Heinemann, London.
6. Sasson, D. (1987) *Italy*, Routledge & Kegan Paul, London.
7. Pinto, D. (ed) (1981) *Contemporary Italian Sociology: A Reader*, Cambridge University Press, Cambridge.
8. Robb, J.H. (1986) 'The Italian Health Service: Slow revolution or permanent crisis?' *Social Science and Medicine*, 22, 6, pp. 619–27.
9. Parry-Jones, W. (1972) *The Trade in Lunacy*, Routledge & Kegan Paul, London.
10. A good historical account of intervention methods is provided in: Baruch, J., Treacher, A. (1978) *Psychiatry Observed*, Macmillan, London.
11. Jones, K. (1972) *The History of the Mental Health Services*, Routledge & Kegan Paul, London.
12. DHSS, *Health and Personal Social Services Statistics, 1984, 1987*, HMSO, London.
13. Jones, M. (1952) *Social Psychiatry*, Tavistock, London. Clark, D. (1964) *Administrative Therapy*, Tavistock, London.
14. Guntrip, H. (1971) *Psychoanalytic Theory, Therapy and the Self*, Hogarth Press, London (this book provides a good summary of what has become known as the British psychoanalytical school); Skinner, B.F. (1972) *Beyond Freedom and Dignity*, Pelican, Harmondsworth.
15. Laing, R.D. (1960) *The Divided Self*, Tavistock, London; Laing, R.D. (1971) *The Politics of the Family*, Tavistock, London; Cooper, D. (1967) *Anti-Psychiatry*, Penguin, Harmondsworth.
16. Clare, A. (1978) *Psychiatry in Dissent*, Tavistock, London; British Association of Social Workers (1977) *Mental Health Crisis Services: A New Philosophy*, BASW Publications, London.

17. See Ramon, S. (1985) *Psychiatry in Britain: Meaning and Policy*, Croom Helm, Chapters 6 and 8, and the second report of the House of Commons Social Services Committee on Community Care, published by HMSO, January 1985.

18. Manacorda, A., Montella, V. (1977) *La Nuova Psichiatria in Italia*, Feltrinelli Economica, Milan.

19. Basaglia, F. (1968) *L'Istituzione Negata*, Einaudi, Milan.

20. Casagrande, D. et al. (1972) 'Lettera di congedo dall'ospedale', in Basaglia, F., Tranchina, P. (ed) (1980) *Autobiografia di un Movimento 1961–1979*, Amministrazione di Arezzo, pp. 162–5.

21. The first congress of *Psichiatria Democratica* took place in Arezzo, 24–6 September 1967. Apart from the collection mentioned in ref. 20, the group publishes a bi-monthly journal (*Fogli di Informazione*). A relatively recent summary of the issues it is concerned with appears in the volume: Crepet, P. et al. (ed) (1983) *Fra Regole e Utopia*, Cooperativa Editoriale Psichiatria Democratica.

22. A recent translation of F. Basaglia's major writings has appeared in: Scheper Hughes, N., Lovell, A. (1987) *In and Out of Psychiatry*, Columbia University Press, New York.

23. Tansella, M. et al. (1986) 'The Italian Psychiatric Reform: Some Quantitative Evidence', *International Journal of Social Psychiatry*.

24. Sayce, L. (1987) 'Overview of British CMHCs', annual conference of the National Unit for Psychiatric Research and Development, pp. 2–5.

25. See ref. 23.

26. DHSS, *Health and Personal Social Services Statistics, 1985*, HMSO, London.

27. See ref. 23 above.

28. Teresini, L., Trebiancini, M. (1985) 'I servizi territoriali costano meno del manicomio: recerca comparate sulla spesa psichiatrica delle quattro provincie del Friuli-Venezia Guilia', *Fogli di Informazione*, 111, pp. 1–13.

29. *The Mental Health Amendments Act, 1983*, HMSO, London. For a full exposition of the Act, see Gostin, L. (1983) *The Mental Health Act 1983: A Guide*, MIND Publications, London.

30. Rogers, A. (1987) *A Place of Safety*, MIND Publications, London.

31. Gostin, L. (1976) *A Human Condition*, MIND Publications, Leeds.

32. See the 1985 report from the Social Services Committee on the care of the adult mentally ill.

33. Basaglia, F. (1980) 'Problems of Law and Psychiatry', *International Journal of Law and Psychiatry*, 3, 3, pp. 17–37.

34. Censis (1985) *Psichiatria: Il dopo 180*, vol. XXI, 8, speciale estate, Rome.

35. Cravedi, B. (1982) 'Analisi comparativa delle proposte relative alla psichiatria', *Salute e Territorio*, 25, pp. 40–2.

36. Jones, K. (1985) 'Understanding the Italian Experience', *British Journal of Psychiatry*, 146, pp. 341–7.

Part I

The Experience of
Psychiatry in Transition

Editor's Introduction

This first part describes the experiences of the two psychiatric systems for the users at different stages and places within these frameworks: the authors look at what being a user means for individuals (Davis, Mangen); what may happen to a person in a mental distress crisis (Brangwyn, Dell'Acqua); after a long period of hospitalization (Mangen, Henry); when the user is a woman, a member of an ethnic minority, of a marginal group, or when they are being put in a special hospital-prison (Pilgrim, Del Giudice). Lack of hope and lack of self-respect are expressed by the users who continue to define themselves via the demands of others (Davis, Selig, Cogliati).

We get also the sense of what may happen to the professionals involved: their marginalization and complicity in British society (Jenner); their emphasis on availability and taking responsibility (Brangwyn, Dell'Acqua); their need, wish and ability to move from the level of working only with individuals to working with the collective too (Canosa, Holland, Salvi). Although left unsaid, the personal costs of the type of professional involvement advocated here by both British and Italian workers must be very high.

The text gives us some indications of what the transition may mean: on the one hand it implies fear of and a reality of neglect (Davis), continuous imposition at every level of living because 'we know what is best for you' (Mangen), and justification of harm in the name of liberalism and tolerance (Selig). For a minority it implies also total expulsion from society (Pilgrim, Del Giudice).

On the other hand it can signify the beginning of being seen, heard and validated (Giannichedda, Davis, Holland, Salvi, Cogliati, Dell'Acqua). This beginning is followed by the professionals being there consistently and constantly (Brangwyn, Dell'Acqua, Salvi), a general acceptance that one's psychiatric symptomatology is a reflection of being stuck rather than of being ill for good, the demonstration of respect and yet the ability to maintain constraints (see Dell'Acqua and Mezzina's description of how compulsory admission is handled in an open local service). Taking a person seriously means also being with them on holiday at the seaside (Canosa), encouraging them to have a bank account (Henry), as well as encouraging them to take part in local social action (Holland, Giannichedda, Salvi).

Today's state of transition implies also making space for new voices to be heard (Davis, Giannichedda, Selig, Cogliati, Holland), and experimenting with services' structures and content (Henry). Above all it means taking informed risks with oneself as a worker, with one's team, encouraging one's clients and the public too to do so (Del Giudice).

Three central components come out of these descriptions and analysis:

- One by one, the contributions attest to the untapped human potential of users who have been given up in the near past as 'chronic patients'. The potential is reflected at the levels of intellectual, social and affective performance. The shared approach of all authors is to see users as people with problems, rather than as bearers of diagnostic entities.

- The professionals' ability to discover and encourage the hitherto untapped potential in patients depends not on the development of new skills, but on the adoption of a mentality which differs considerably from that of traditional psychiatry. Henry's emphasis on the need to understand better health rather than pathology summarizes the change neatly. The quotation from Basaglia in Giannichedda's text on the price paid by the workers in the process of transition is another aspect that cannot be forgotten, and contributes to our understanding of why it is so difficult for many workers to change their past mentality (Davis, Mangen). In their own ways, the different contributions also outline the type of skills required within the new approach to psychiatry. These are skills of firm, yet unoppressive and supportive presence, of informal yet attentive listening; a high degree of informality and involvement in concrete, daily experiences; not to be flustered by panic; a high level of improvisation and innovation in the use of resources; and the ability to act at both the individual and the collective levels.

- The third element which this section shows to be crucial for the transition is the need for, and the possibility of changing, the general public's approach to mental distress and to people defined as suffering from it. This perspective is exemplified in the work on the integration of children with handicaps (Salvi and Cecchini); in forcing on the public an encounter with long-term residents of a mental hospital (Giannichedda); by organizing women clients into a group which is campaigning for the benefit of others as much as for that of its members (Holland); in changing women's perceptions of their own bodies and sexuality (Cogliati, Petri, Pini), by the readiness of the Italian Constitutional Court to allow offenders with mental distress to live outside the psychiatric prison (Chapter 14), under the supervision of a local mental health service.

The text also shows that with initiative, dedication and pressure, local resources are found in a climate of cuts in welfare spending (Brangwyn), or in relatively poor areas with unsympathetic authorities (Canosa). The outstanding issue is what is the best use of the available resources to meet the double objective of desegregation and reintegration not only of the users of the psychiatric services, but also of the professionals and the public.

The similarity in approach between the British and Italian contributors to this section is considerable. Beginning with sharing the same objectives of de-hospitalization and de-institutionalization, it continues through the emphasis on professionals' attitudes and commitments, the focus on collective involvement, the concern with individuals and the recognition of the need to change society's approach.

The similarities should not mask the differences. For example, the British critique of special hospitals sees the solution in small secure units while in the Italian new practice there is no place for secure provision specifically for the mentally distressed offender: instead it advocates that such people should either be cared for by local mental health services or in an ordinary prison. While in Britain we are encouraging a formal voice for users and take pride in adding to the existing list of formal rights, the Italians are stressing the informal dialogue on a much larger scale than has been attempted so far in Britain.

Significant differences also emerge regarding the structure and focus of services in relation to crisis work and the more general issue of specialized vs generic mental health services. It is hoped that readers will attempt to understand the reasons for the differences before deciding which option makes more sense to them.

Shulamit Ramon

1
Users' Perspectives

ANN DAVIS

Over the last 30 years, marked changes have taken place in the British mental health service. These have had a considerable impact on the lives of people both working in and using mental health provision. Descriptions of these changes and their consequences abound, but they are, in the main, professional and political. Accounts which provide a consumer's perspective are harder to find. They have to be gleaned from articles, autobiographies, radio interviews, newspaper exposés, film and television documentaries. But these are fragments scattered over three decades.[1] They tell us something, but by no means enough, about the way in which those who use mental health provision have been served by it.

From the available fragments we know that the lives and choices of hundreds of thousands of consumers have been profoundly affected by the adoption of 'community care' policies. For some people community care has meant moving from familiarly bleak, routinized living in large wards of mental hospitals into the unknown. For too many, the unknown has revealed itself to be the overcrowded, unsanitary conditions of the most deprived sector of the private rented housing market. In board and lodging houses in inner cities and by the sea, thousands of men and women are living their lives in considerable stress and poverty. Many live below the state's own poverty line as they use their social security benefits to meet housing costs which the government no longer meets in full.

For others, community care means group living in specialist hostels or group homes which can work out well or badly, but from which there is little chance of moving on. Yet others have found themselves living again with members of their family, subject to the strong positive and negative forces inherent in family life.

Despite this movement away from long-term hospital care, the shift to community care policies in Britain has not meant that institutions are no longer major resource holders. Our former, nineteenth century asylums still retain a large proportion of the personnel and services available to those suffering mental distress and disturbance. However, for all but the elderly, such institutions no longer provide the long-term solution of segregation and containment. The expectation of mental health experts is that most consumers will find ways of coping with their difficulties in the context of community or family life. The only readily available support on offer in the community is chemical. Other forms of help are at best variable and often non-existent. Hospital beds are usually offered as a last resort and so, for some consumers, success is now measured by time between admissions:

> Like many patients I have a return ticket to psychiatric hospital. I'm not boasting or complaining and it does get better. My stays are getting shorter and there are longer periods between.[2]

Central and local government and mental health professionals caught up in the changes of the last 30 years have systematically ignored consumers' perspectives. They have rarely surveyed or researched consumers' views and experiences or involved consumers in planning and service provision. Yet this lack of interest in the consumer's perspective has not prevented both professionals' and politicians' claims that the changes they advocate are in the 'best interests' of consumers and their families.

Professional and political accounts of change suggest that one of the central concerns of the state and mental health employees has been to improve consumers' experiences of the service. One of the dominant rationales for change in both government statements of intent and professional accounts of new therapeutic directions is that consumers will benefit. The contraction of large psychiatric hospitals and the emphasis on locating care and treatment in 'the community' has been continuously promoted as a less stigmatized and more flexible response to consumers' needs.

The vivid imagery used by Enoch Powell in 1961 conjured up a vision of a new era of provision which would remove from the lives of users and their communities the blight of state psychiatric hospitals – 'isolated, majestic, imperious ... rising unmistakeable and daunting out of the countryside'.[3] To live without the fear of incarceration in such institutions could only be of benefit to any person suffering mental distress, he argued.

The reality which many consumers experienced in the wake of the first contractions of psychiatric hospitals fell far short of this vision.

The promise of community-based support and treatment remained just that. Throughout the country people suffering mental distress still had to turn to the specialist institutions for a response to their difficulties. At the same time those who had spent a large part of their adult lives as inmates of psychiatric hospitals found their bags being packed for evacuation.

The expectation was that they would manage in the outside world. Some hospitals developed rehabilitation programmes to help patients make the transition. But there was no uniform approach. In the worst situations, consumers were offered very little.

A psychiatric social worker in North Wales during the 1960s found that the 'rehabilitation programme' being pursued by his local psychiatric hospital meant that:

> patients were simply thrown out of the hospital without preparation. Buses and coaches collected them and they were crammed into boarding houses, dumped on landladies. One group of patients were placed with a woman whose own children were in care. It was a travesty of a service for vulnerable, frightened people.[4]

While events like this sometimes hit the headlines of the local and national press, government attention was firmly focused elsewhere. It was the poor quality care, neglect and ill-treatment suffered by patients in mental illness hospitals which were highlighted in a stream of official public and local enquiries in the late 1960s and early 1970s.[5] Those ex-inmates trying to reestablish their lives in isolated, poverty-stricken conditions in the community found their plight virtually ignored by state bodies. Sometimes the fate of these consumers was thrust under the noses of politicians or mental health professionals. When this happened the official response tended to be that unfortunately they were carrying some of the 'costs' of change, but were still 'lucky' to have escaped the damaging effects of institutionalization.

By the mid 1970s, the message was clear. Whatever the experiences of consumers and their families, those developing policy were convinced that community care held the key to the future. In 1975 the publication of *Better Services for the Mentally Ill* (which contains objectives still held to be central to policy and provision in Britain) reiterated the theme of consumer advantage.

Better Services describes the 'new pattern of services' based on a shift to community provision and 'multi-professional teamwork' as being 'in the patient's best interest'. It is argued that such an approach enables mental health professionals 'to identify and respond to widely varying individual needs for care and support'[6] and at the same time provides opportunities for 'the individual and his family to be made to feel that they themselves have a positive contribution to make to the whole process'.[7]

This was, and is, pure speculation. No evidence was available, or had been sought, to support such claims. What is more they were made at a time when radical reorganization of the health and social services had effectively weakened the organizational basis of a co-ordinated, multi-professional mental health service. This, together with public expenditure restraint, seemed bound to undermine the already precarious foundation of the 'new pattern of services'.

At no stage during these first two decades of change was serious attention paid to the relationship between consumers and professionals in the 'new pattern' of services. The hierarchical medical model of care and treatment which was so often described as an inherent feature of psychiatric institutions was attacked in anti-institutional literature. These attacks echoed earlier critiques developed as part of the therapeutic community movement. Essentially staff–patient relationships emanating from this model were seen as stifling patient growth and development and reinforcing staff power. However the implicit assumption in the 1960s and 1970s seemed to be that the relocation of services would automatically change this approach to consumers. It was as if transplanting provision from a mental hospital to a psychiatric clinic, day hospital or unit located in a general hospital was all that was needed radically to change the relationship between consumers and professionals.

Of course this has not proved to be the case, as many consumers have discovered. It needed more than a change of building to alter the way in which mental health professionals worked with their 'clients' and 'patients'. Most medical, nursing and social services staff retained in their hearts and minds the notion of consumers as damaged individuals who needed advice and management. Professional preoccupations with the difficulties, problems and 'weaknesses' of consumers rendered them passive recipients of services controlled by professionals who decided what was 'best'. The consequence for consumers has been that most community-based provision has replicated the all too familiar relationships of institutional life. Such relationships serve to confirm the worst fears that consumers have about themselves. They focus on helplessness and inability and so sap confidence and a sense of self.

Recognizing the basis of such relationships does not always help. Consumers can still feel trapped or damaged. In the words of a woman in her mid-fifties, who shared with me her views on the staff who had cared for her for years in a psychiatric hospital:

> They meant well, don't get me wrong. I'm not criticizing them. They thought it was all for the best, for our own good, but they treated us like children. They made your mind up for you and you stopped thinking for yourself. They said we could not be expected to cope with the ups and downs of life. It did me no good, I lost confidence altogether.[8]

The changes we have witnessed in the British mental health services have not eradicated psychiatric institutions, or their traditional approach to consumers. The changes have not been informed by consumers' views, ideas and participation. Yet in the 1980s the message that the scale and direction of change is in the best interests of consumers is louder and clearer than ever.

Care in the Community, a consultative document from the government published at the beginning of the 1980s, opens with the claim:

> Most people who need long-term care can and should be looked after in the community. This is what most of them want for themselves and what those responsible for their care believe to be best.[9]

This happy coincidence of consumer and professional preference for current policies has become a taken-for-granted fact of both professional and political debate on mental health provision. But it is no more than assertion, based on an over-simplified claim that there is a choice for consumers between bad (institutional) responses and good (community) responses. Reality is much more complex for those suffering mental distress and their families. Too many people in the 1980s who are drawn into mental health provision are as neglected, discounted, abused and ignored, as consumers of earlier periods.[10] The individualized, flexible responses of multidisciplinary teams do not often materialize outside of official reports. Consumers usually experience disjointed and confusing encounters, over which they feel they have little control:

> I went to see my doctor when I was 15 and experiencing out-of-body sensations. I was given phenobarbitone. I saw him again after the birth of my first baby when I was suffering from post-natal depression. I was given tranquillizers and told I was an irresponsible student. I'd got myself into this mess and must get myself out of it. This put me off going to see a doctor for several years.

A social worker came round once but wasn't much help. Two and a half years ago, I went to see a GP and was prescribed Valium and referred to out-patients' to see a psychiatrist. I was visited three times by a community psychiatric nurse who was no help at all. He kept using platitudes like 'Look on the bright side.' I went back to see my doctor who wouldn't see me unless my husband was there. I was very depressed and the doctor said he couldn't handle me.[11]

It is by not listening and learning from these kind of experiences that politicians and mental health professionals can continue to talk about a reality that consumers do not recognize: an official reality that is blind to the impact that under-resourced and unreliable mental health services are having on the lives of consumers and their families.

But are times changing? In 1985 came the first acknowledgement in an official report that 'Too little attention has been paid in the past to the views of those most closely affected by the policy of community care'.[12] Two paragraphs on consumers' views in the *Social Services Committee Report on Community Care*, with special reference to adult mentally ill and mentally handicapped people, is little enough but it marks a beginning, one which the current government has declared it wishes to develop further.[13] This arrival of consumer perspectives onto the political agenda is the outcome of at least three distinct influences. First, consumerism. For nearly a decade now British governments have been concerned to roll back state welfare provision and promote private welfare activity. In arguing its case for a 'mixed economy of welfare' government representatives have claimed that it will give consumers a better deal. The NHS is being exhorted not only to 'privatize' parts of its provision but to establish quality assurance – all in the interest of consumers. In such a climate consumer views have become an important measure of successful change.

Second, the pressure groups which have over many years become part of the mental health scene, such as MIND (National Association of Mental Health) and the National Schizophrenia Fellowship, have regularly published and promoted consumers' and relatives' views of services they have received. These views have covered a wide range of issues, from the civil liberties of detained patients to the impact on relatives of hospital closure. They amount to a substantial body of evidence on the failure of the services to engage with the views of consumers and their relatives.

Finally, there has been a visible increase in the activities of consumer organizations during the 1980s. Some have focused on particular issues such as the effects of tranquillizers and have worked to support members withdrawing from their use of such drugs. Others, such as the Campaign Against Psychiatric Oppression, which sees psychiatric treatment as a means of control and oppression, locate victims of psychiatry alongside other oppressed groups and argue that they must engage with them in collective action in order to change their situation.[14]

In 1985 the first national network for consumers of the psychiatric services, 'Survivors Speak Out', began. This group is concerned to provide a means for consumers to meet and share information, views, experiences and ideas for changing the services they receive. This initiative aims to extend the work of self-advocacy groups in Britain. At its first national conference in September 1987, it established itself as an important forum for supporting consumers' views and action in mental health services.

Whatever the reasons for the recent acknowledgement in government circles of the importance of consumers' views, little evidence exists that it has percolated through to the majority of mental health professionals. There have been no substantial developments in either mental health research or practice which indicate a willingness to work with consumers in planning, developing, providing and managing mental health services. The few projects which have taken this path, against the mainstream of professional opinion, show just what the gains might be for consumers and workers alike.

In 1983 a team of social services social workers in Coventry set up a Crisis Intervention Service (CIS) which offered an alternative to hospitalization for people deemed by psychiatrists to be in crisis. The social workers were concerned to ensure that consumers' perspectives informed the development of the service. They therefore asked their first 50 consumers to share their views of the help they had been offered. As part of this exercise consumers were asked to compare what they had gained from the time-limited intervention offered by this service with their previous experience of psychiatric care and treatment. It was clear that the relationship established with service workers was often experienced as a partnership of great value.

The presence of social workers rather than psychiatrists put a perspective on my problems making me realise I was not abnormal, just mixed up. The difference between psychiatrists and social workers is that the social workers made me face up to my own problems and realise that I was the one who would solve them. This is because social workers are in effect 'real people' whereas psychiatrists are 'doctors' ... [and] the onus is on the doctor to cure.

[It's] better than hospital where I was pumped with drugs for four days. CIS is concerned with what's been happening after and this is helpful.

[Workers] don't adopt a 'holier than thou' attitude, which makes it easier to open up about problems. CIS turned what shouldn't have happened into the best thing that could have happened.[15]

It is feedback of this kind from consumers which workers in the Coventry service have found invaluable in reviewing and developing their practice and the project. Such exchanges are vital to any service concerned to meet the needs of individuals suffering crises and distress.

However before they can begin to listen to consumers many mental health professionals will need to examine the assumptions they make about those who use their services. The act of labelling an individual as 'suitable' for mental health provision involves judgements about the 'irrationality' or 'madness' of that individual. These judgements all too often result in a denial by professionals that any opinion or view expressed by a consumer can be valid. As a result consumer perspectives are not accepted as pertinent to assessing and developing a service. Consumer participation in management and service delivery is dismissed as unrealistic. The distance between consumers and professionals is maintained. The North Derbyshire Mental Health Services Project, described in Chapter 19 by Rick Hennelly, is unique in challenging this distance and the structures which maintain it.

It is a fundamental change in the hearts and minds of those working in our mental health services that has been missing over the last three decades. There have been all too few attempts to work with consumers on their difficulties and those of the services. Such work can take a variety of forms and can address itself to a number of issues. It can, for example, be directed at making services more accessible to those who might benefit from them. Consumers know a great deal about what is of value in a particular service. When consumers' views are taken account of, that service can increase its relevance to, and use by, others.

Consumers' 'perceptive and imaginative'[16] perspectives can and should inform joint work in planning as well as managing services. The recognition that consumers are a 'source of wisdom'[17] which needs to be tapped for the benefit of all those involved in our mental health services is long overdue.

References

1. Brandon, D. (1981) *Voices of Experience: Consumer Perspectives of*

Psychiatric Treatment, MIND Publications, London.

2. *Experiences of a Changing Kind: Adult Education in Psychiatric Hospitals and Day Centres* (1985) MIND and Workers Education Association, London.

3. *Co-ordination or Chaos? The Rundown of Psychiatric Hospitals*, MIND (1974) report no. 13, London.

4. Davies, N. (1979) 'Well, then I met these lunatics...', Chapter 5 in Brandon, D., Jordan, B. *Creative Social Work*, Basil Blackwell, Oxford.

5. Beardshaw, V. (1981) *Conscientiousness Objectors at Work: Mental Hospital Nurses, A Case Study*, Social Audit.

6. DHSS (1975) *Better Services for the Mentally Ill*, p. 10, paragraph 1.31.

7. Ibid., p. 10, paragraph 1.32.

8. Davis, A., Muir, L. (1984) 'Working with Volunteers and Self-Help Groups', Chapter 13 in M.R. Olsen (ed) *Social Work and Mental Health: A Guide for the Approved Social Worker*, Tavistock, London, p. 161.

9. DHSS (1981) *Care in the Community: A Consultative Document*, HMSO.

10. Kay, A., Legg, C. (1968) *Discharge to the Community: A Review of Housing and Support in London for People Leaving Psychiatric Care*, Housing Research Group, The City University.

11. Dyer, L. (1985) *Wrong End of the Telescope*, MIND Publications, London, p. 8.

12. DHSS (1985) *Community Care with special reference to adult mentally ill and mentally handicapped people*, Second Report from the Social Services Select Committee, 1984–5 session, HMSO.

13. DHSS (1985) Government Response to the Second Report from the Social Services Committee 1984–5 session, ibid.

14. CAPO (1985) *Introduction to the Manifesto*.

15. Davis, A., Newton, S., Smith, D. (1985) 'Coventry Crisis Intervention Team: The Consumers' View', *Social Services Research*, vol. 14, no. 1.

16. Fisher, M., Newton, C., Sainsbury E. (1984) *Mental Health Social Work Observed*, Allen & Unwin, London.

17. Brandon, D. (1981) *Voices of Experience*.

2

A Future of Social Invisibility

MARIA GRAZIA GIANNICHEDDA

At the beginning of the 1970s the process of transforming psychiatry moved beyond the boundaries of 'exemplary experiences' to the national level. This brought into focus the issues related to listening and attending to the voice of the patient in the ongoing debate of the alternatives to the total institution. The power and the right of patients to participate in this debate became one of the major themes in the encounter between the two lines of reform which by then had begun to be delineated: de-hospitalization, that is the administrative reduction of psychiatric institutions; and de-institutionalization. The latter entails a radical review of the relationship between those offering treatment and those being treated on the one hand and between psychiatric institutions and society on the other.

The passing of Law 180 clarified the conflict between these two ideas for reform but in no way resolved it. Today both solutions coexist in Italy; they present two different accounts of the transition from mental hospitals to district services, and two different models of community psychiatric practice. The patient's freedom and the importance of his/her wishes is fundamentally different in the two cases. Similarly, their respective cultures of mental illness and health are transmitted to society and to the users themselves in a fundamentally different way. In one case, as we shall see, the transformation of psychiatry has resulted in its users achieving some form of organized, public expression and a certain level of autonomy in managing their own problems. In the other case, calls from family associations (which have been formed to request new kinds of internment) sometimes accompany the silence, isolation and impotence of the users.

In this respect, the current situation in Italian psychiatry confirms what was central to the thinking put forward by the group surrounding Franco and Franca Basaglia – the culture of the demand reflects the culture of the response and the former is channelled and modelled by the latter. The silence or the requests of the users and of society need also to be understood in relation to the implicit and explicit teaching given by psychiatric institutions in all their forms.

There are certain indicators which will point to a service's political aims and operational choices, rather than the culture of its users and society. These indicators are, first, the degree to which society accepts patients and, second, the degree to which patients accept that their suffering is related to their own problems of communicating with others and their own experience of living. Likewise, the rejection of patients and their institutionalized expressions of suffering point primarily to the extent to which the importance of asylum culture is underestimated by reformers and politicians who perceive the reform as a mere administrative exercise which involves only those who are 'fit for work'.

The following analysis will review the various orientations of responses from psychiatric institutions. Of course, this does not mean that autonomous spaces for expression and culture do not exist outside institutions; but we need to emphasize that institutions should take cultural and political responsibility for the type of orientation chosen on behalf of users and society. 'Opening the institution is not opening the door, it is opening one's mind when faced with a sick person.'[1]

When psychiatric hospitals initiate the relationship between patients who go out and the town which they visit it is like a dialogue between deaf people or between worlds which speak strange and different languages. On the one hand there is the patient who is locked into his/her suffering and institutional language; on the other, there is a town which has never known real patients and which has only learnt about the dangerousness and incomprehensibility of their illness.

Psychiatric workers are the only intermediaries in this relationship. Their attitude during this stage will be crucial to the future development of any community psychiatric practice.

The de-institutionalization experiences which took place in Italy in the early 1970s and which modelled themselves on the experiment undertaken by the therapeutic community of the Gorizia psychiatric hospital chose to act simultaneously on the institutions, the patients and the public. As soon as the doors of the psychiatric hospital were opened, the relationship with the outside world began. Discussions were taking place between doctors, nurses and patients on the organization of institutional life, and negotiations were being held with administrators on resources. Patients went out and the public was invited inside to parties, meetings and cultural events.

In all the examples where this style of operating was chosen, the first stage brought with it different levels of conflict both inside and outside.

> I know that you experienced serious personal crises when your work
> was being discussed, when you were no longer in authority over
> patients, and when you understood that patients had the same rights
> as you.[2]

> We turned suffering from the mental hospital out onto the streets, and
> this led the town to discover its own suffering which was codified in
> other separate institutions.[3]

These two levels of conflict, one inside concerning patients' wishes, the
other outside concerning the presence of patients in the town, were the
most difficult ones in the experiment. Yet they were probably the most
productive facets. As the work progressed gradually, it became
increasingly apparent that identifying the boundary between these
conflicts was both ambiguous and difficult. The hospital's management
group had to find a balance between searching for consensus as opposed to
new forms of oppression which denied a patient's individuality. It had
to take account of security measures, measures to encourage responsibility
and measures to ensure tolerance.

> We are living on experience to which we hold the key, and we are
> responsible for relationships which should always be open, and we
> must ensure that they remain open, not closed.[4]

This way of operating tended to encourage conflicts to be brought out
into the open and to change them into opportunities for collective
consciousness-raising. At the same time, this 'conflict tuition' changed
psychiatric problems from being fringe problems – and as such exclusive
to professionals and administrators in the field – into social problems
which involved the general public, the media, other institutions and
social movements. This was possible because the image of the patient
who went around the town was not hidden or minimized, but on the
contrary was emphasized. Inmates spoke publicly, discussed matters
from a personal point of view – such as their right to live, work, consume
and speak out. They sought solidarity with other members of the public
who were experiencing similar conditions of disadvantage.

The transition from the psychiatric hospital to a district service
which was carried out in this way produced significant results
concerning the internal relationships within the service and its
relationship with society in general. In the case of the first, ex-patients

and new users were able to strengthen their position within the structure in their dealings with workers, because they had built for themselves a small, social space on the outside. In addition, because they were able to use language which was different from that of the institution, they were able to make themselves heard. This protected patients (partially at least) from the risk of their expressions being interpreted only according to the service's restricting codes.

In fact when patients are able to express themselves not only inside the institutional or family context but also to other individuals and even in public, and when they are able to speak about the significance of not only their own personal experiences but also that of others, it is less easy for their words to be abruptly disregarded as 'sick' words, which acquire meaning only in relation to the code of illness. It also becomes possible for patients to be responsible for their own words and actions. This brings us to the second result of preventing patients being cast into the social role of the 'psychiatrized'. This role leads them to speak only about themselves or on their own behalf, and hence to continue to be disregarded as a 'minority interest'. As we shall see, in some cases, users of the psychiatric service succeeded in promoting a much wider debate about the needs of all individuals who for various reasons end up on the margins of society and about the meaning of this condition.

The patient's individualized presence was not easily accepted either inside or outside the institution. It was not even accepted in those places where the struggle to achieve this was more intense and informed. In fact this presence would require a cultural and organizational change, not only of psychiatric services but of all institutions, and would also require a change in society's dominant values. These processes of adaptation would enable those who suffer in their social experience to speak out. In fact, they are a necessary and central condition, if society is to be able to make adequate provision for life without psychiatric hospitals. Without these processes, the need for psychiatric hospitals will re-emerge and will assume tougher, more cynical characteristics than before.

This will be evident if we look at those places in Italy, and the US in particular, where a consistent reduction in psychiatric treatment has taken place on the grounds of administrative rationalization. In these cases, when patients are imposed on the town without apparent conflict and also without 'explanations' or support, when the city life is forced on patients without their being able to enjoy the rights and duties of citizenship, then patients experience extreme social rejection. At the same time the activists among them develop forms of closed shop. This type of solution, which provides neither meaning nor relationships between society and ex-patients, has produced an end to the game, in which it is the weakest who are the most vulnerable, despite the fact that their rights have been formally confirmed.

'For Us, the Street is a Factory of Fate'⁵

How can we prevent the kind of fate which means that discharged patients – whether long-term or new – tend to drift into the most marginal areas of society and do not succeed in leaving them? There is a fundamental difference between those who, in the course of their illness, have been able to strengthen their personal life and social role, and those who have experienced their illness shut away by the illness/therapy ideology in a space separated by the service. In the second case, even though the disorder may have passed, the individual's social and subjective isolation will not have changed, s/he will easily be weakened and lose the struggle to find a space for living. In the first case, however, the individual's experience of suffering becomes an opportunity for confronting other people and for social participation. Then the discovery or creation of new forms of organization and culture can offer him/her both practical solutions to life and a new self-image, which will support him/her in an uncertain future.

Inside the psychiatric service this sort of encouragement for the user to take responsibility is supported by various aspects of the organization. In the community mental health centre no place is prohibited to users, nor designated for them alone (except, of course, the bedrooms which are theirs full time). Similarly the medicine cupboard is open. Individual consultations with workers (including doctors) take place in communal areas which from time to time can be used privately by whoever requires it. Everybody is allowed to use the telephone and to be present at meetings, including those of staff. There are no locations in which users alone participate because it was decided not to restrict their space at any one time.

However, there are structures which are managed exclusively by users. These structures vary according to their historical, geographical and cultural context: committees for housing, social problems, women's groups, groups for young users with similar problems and so on. Of all these structures, which are usually shortlived according to whether or not there are active people within the service, or people with serious problems, two have survived from the outset; both are also widespread and co-ordinated at national level. They provide examples of the particular form of expression which users in Italy found useful throughout the processes designed to change psychiatric practice.

The first of these was created to deal with work problems and belongs to the first stage of de-institutionalization. The second is more recent, and deals with problems of communication for users concerning the political status and living conditions of those who live on the fringes of society.

The first example is the work co-operatives based on the one created in Trieste by a small group of about 30 psychiatric patients who undertook hospital cleaning work and gardening work. Under the old institutional system, this had been called occupational therapy. Within the co-operative it became work which was paid by the local administration. There are currently 65 co-operatives of this type in Italy with about 2,000 associates. They have been re-aligned into the National Co-ordinating Body for Co-operatives against Marginalization, whose headquarters are in Turin. Over time these co-operatives have admitted associates such as the physically handicapped, drug addicts, ex-prisoners and 'ordinary' unemployed people. Despite many difficulties these structures have now entered the free market but have neither been able nor have wanted to hide their suffering and its problematic relation with the ideology of productivity. The political identity of these structures was created precisely by the difficulties in reconciling work, production and the market to people, health and the quality of life and relationships; and the problem of 'adapting work and the market place to man while the converse has always been true' – as one of the founder members of the co-ordinating body said during the first of two national conferences which they have held.

In this way these co-operatives have firstly instituted a series of innovations at the work organization level, regarding distribution of tasks, organization structure, control of time, training, which would merit detailed analysis elsewhere. Second, they have undertaken to defend the rights of those who are socially sick or deviant when confronted by the psychiatric, welfare and the legal systems. In this sense they have developed into structures which are different from 'normal' workplaces but which are not welfare structures or are there just to protect rights. This 'spurious' identity, which in the initial stages was a weakness when they needed to assert themselves in the labour market and the political world, is nowadays a strength, which gives these co-operatives the authority to express themselves on social services and on problems concerning the quality of life and work. In fact, these patients who work on the one hand explode the myth of the patient who is unproductive. On the other hand they criticize work as a value in itself, and support a culture of individual expression which aims to change the meaning of work itself.

The subjective expression of suffering, the image of the world which conditions the suffering, is the theme of the second type of structure created in Italy by users of the psychiatric services.

These take the form of various cultural associations which have different names (in Rome, Trieste, Bari, Venice and Turin they are called 'Franco Basaglia Associations') and they are beginning to become nationally co-ordinated bodies. These structures are managed by users, ex-users and professionals. They have created various types of cultural workshops: poetry, drama, music, painting, video production, sporting and tourist activities. Like all associations, they have access to public funding because of their work programmes or services to society and they make use of both consultants from related fields of expertise (actors, directors, poets etc.) and psychiatric workers. In this case also, the plan is to avoid patients becoming introverted into their own condition, whether it be illness, youth or marginality, by creating spaces for everybody (festivals, open-air discotheques, meetings and parties); also the fact that marginal languages are not intercommunicative is borne in mind.

So far the material products of these associations are a new attempt to link youth culture to classical forms of culture popular with older people. The reason they are so successful in the cultural arena is because of their originality. A catalogue of the materials and organizational prototypes produced by these organizations is currently being prepared. This will form part of a programme to co-ordinate similar associations which were created for drug addicts and young marginals.

Against a Future of Social Invisibility

Today the co-operatives and associations mentioned above are part of a larger network which deals with psychiatric problems, and various users take part in them: i.e. the Association for Struggle Against Mental Illness, the Association for Freedom From the Need for Prisons and Total Institutions, many local committees For the Application of Law 180, and several relatives' associations who oppose the reopening of mental hospitals. The weight of these bodies in the social and political life, in the debate on psychiatric reform, has been significant in recent years but very hotly contested. Stereotypes of the madman who is 'dangerous, incomprehensible, asocial' or who is 'an idiot, fragile, unproductive' have often been put forward after the passing of Law 180, especially by relatives' associations who, unlike those mentioned above, have organized the lobby for the construction of new forms of internment for mental patients and drug addicts.

The confrontation between the two groups is apparently about tidying up the legal and institutional position, but in fact the issues at stake go a lot deeper.

The groups lobbying for a return to internment are proposing and requesting more than just a few 'protected' institutions. They want to see a return to the principle of authority – of the family and of science – where the weak are invalidated by professional custody, the reasons for suffering are stifled and the 'cure' is considered achieved only when the patient returns to 'normality'.

For their part, user associations do not opt merely for space and regulation within the services or with regard to psychiatry. They are organized against a future of social invisibility which was built in the past for them by the walls of psychiatric hospitals. This invisibility is reintroduced by dominant social values and the rules of the social game. But the aim of these associations is an ambitious one: the utopia of a space and a meaning in society and history.

This ambition has certainly had the effect of rousing curiosity if not solidarity, and of giving rise to disagreement, rather than consensus. Sometimes people cannot comprehend it, or they reject it, especially those who are willing to offer tolerance and 'good' services while at the same time defending their own power and knowledge. But this ambition has also been the strength of these users' bodies; it has enabled them to survive all the difficulties and to continue to exist as a positive voice.

A discharged long-term patient can die of neglect in a tolerant but inattentive city. This encapsulates both the real and figurative future for a psychiatric user in post-industrial society. Users in Italy have begun to organize against this reality and against this type of future.

References

1. Basaglia, F. (1979) *La Libertà è Terapeutica?* Feltrinelli, Milan, p. 44.
2. Ibid.
3. Ibid., p. 39.
4. Ibid., p. 43.
5. Ibid.

3

Constructing a Crisis-focused Social Service

GILL BRANGWYN

'What', said the consultant psychiatrist, peering through the window, 'is that unicorn doing in the flower bed?' 'It's a statue made by two of the staff – it symbolizes imagination and hope – we want the Centre to stand for that in the minds of the people who come here.' 'Hmm ... symbols won't be much use to you when they try to hang themselves from the balcony. How do you get someone a bed here?'

This sort of conversation is not uncommon at the Lansdowne Lane Community Mental Health Centre which will be described below, as an example of a recent development in response to mental distress crisis.

There are several units in Britain presently offering a mental health crisis intervention service that is similar to that offered at Lansdowne Lane. The first such unit was initiated by social workers and psychiatrists at the Napsbury hospital in 1974.[1] Despite its success in the reduction of first admissions its method of work remains hardly used elsewhere. However, almost all of the existing crisis intervention units are allied to psychiatric hospitals: their funding, admissions, treatment and future are closely linked to the health service power structure. Others, non-statutory agencies, such as the Samaritans, have been operating a crisis intervention service since their inception.

Lansdowne Lane Residential and Community Mental Health Centre, where the conversation quoted above took place, is in Charlton, a pleasant suburban village in the south-east London Borough of Greenwich. The centre, financed, managed and staffed entirely by Greenwich Social Services Department, serves the whole borough – a population of 209,000 people. The borough is a large one, encompassing considerable social and economic diversity. There are increasing numbers of African, Afro-Caribbean and Asian people in the borough. The local government of the area is managed by its Council which is Labour controlled at the time of writing.

The borough has a broad based mental distress service; two general hospitals whose workers provide 'emergency', in-patient and out-patient community-based and day hospital care for a limited number of designated 'psychiatric patients', five area teams of field social workers, three day centres (for people with physical or mental health difficulties), a limited number of domiciliary support workers (home helps, family aides, meals on wheels); an 'out of hours' social work team all of whom are experienced in dealing with mental health problems.

Provision for a mental health service in the borough has been piecemeal and has not benefited from any co-ordinated planning with local statutory health and voluntary bodies, until relatively recently. The need to plan mental health services in an organized way, together with other statutory and voluntary health and social care agencies, became a matter of urgency when the regional health authority, in line with government intentions to run down large mental hospitals and introduce mental health care into 'the community', announced in 1984 the necessity for the district health authority to become 'self-sufficient' in terms of mental health care within the next ten years. This meant that the large mental hospitals in an adjacent borough would no longer be available to Greenwich residents. Since this was where almost all the borough's long- and medium-term patients were treated, it was clear that alternative facilities in Greenwich would have to be made available and with some urgency.

Meanwhile, plans begun many years before for use of the social services department's new 'hostel for the mentally disturbed' continued. These were fraught by fury in the surrounding community who felt that they had a 'loony bin' sneaked upon them by the council and complained of not being consulted on the hostel's use. The collective ire was eventually reduced by the extreme slowness of the building's completion and the removal to other parts of the borough of the main opponents to the scheme. The council meanwhile was being pressed by other sections of the population to provide more services for the mentally and physically disabled. The continued commitment and personal energy of members of the local voluntary mental health group, the chair of the social services committee and a small group of health and social services personnel was needed to keep the building for mental health services. Ideas varied as to its actual use. It is a large institutional building reflecting 1970s ideas on facilities for the 'mentally disturbed' rather than present-day views.

The social services department, in consultation with health service colleagues and service users, finally came to the conclusion that the major areas of need in their immediate provisions for mental health were to provide long-term residential support for persons with a 'chronic' history of mental health difficulties, and a crisis intervention service, also with a residential component, to deal with mental health emergencies which the existing services felt unable or unsuited to deal with. It was decided to use the almost completed 'hostel for the mentally disturbed' for *both* these new ventures! The council made a budget available. In May 1984, eleven years after initial plans for the site were made, I joined the department as officer-in-charge. What I was in charge of was, at that time, an uncompleted unfurnished building, a great number of apparently disconnected papers on thoughts for its use and the instruction to construct and expedite at least two units on the site, staffed and fully operational, preferably by the end of the year!

I came to the post from a long and varied background in statutory and voluntary social work agencies and an academic background in art, social and medical anthropology and social work. A great deal of my experience in social work settings had been in agencies that worked with 'outsiders', people who often terrified themselves, their families and people who tried to help, by their behaviour: expressions of pain and despair. Some of the agencies I had worked in had found ways of responding quickly and practically to contain potentially disastrous situations. Other agencies had dealt effectively with those 'outsiders' who were also 'no-hopers' – who had given up and been given up on by almost everyone else. The whole picture had made me believe that many unlikely things could be accomplished by steady perseverance within a coherent theoretical framework; all should be leavened with a good deal of energy and as much fun as possible for all concerned!

The initial task seemed to be to find out what likely consumers of 'long-term accommodation for the recovered mentally ill' might need, and what a crisis intervention service thought they might need.

Concerning the latter, the issue raised by professionals, service, consumers and family carers was how best to help those people who had become so upset over a life situation, material, social or emotional, that they or their carers felt unable to rely on previous methods of coping. These situations happened at random times, often outside the times when support services were usually available, and proved difficult for the 'identified client', the professional workers, family and wider community to manage. Often the 'identified client' was someone well known to the support services who had tried many different things in the past and they along with the 'client' family and the outside world were feeling frustrated, helpless and exhausted in the face of yet another upset. Other crisis situations which concerned people were extreme emotional upsets caused by social and material situations intermixed; for instance the sudden and often violent break-up of a relationship causing one of the participants to become homeless. Often people presented themselves to the emergency services with such difficulties, but these services – police, casualty departments, fieldwork social services – did not feel able to respond appropriately due to lack of immediately available facilities or extreme pressure of work. The stress provoked by the mounting numbers of such difficulties and the lack of immediate support for them was considerable, despite the regular handling of these problems by the services.

In July 1985 Lansdowne Lane Centre officially opened. The 14 months of preparation had been filled with planning everything – from how many teaspoons were needed; the nature and organization of extensive public consultation; staffing levels required; training for staff; criteria for admission; work whilst in residence; and plans for people going back into the community. Links with other professional and voluntary and community based agencies were initiated. Referrals were taken for the 'long-stay rehabilitation unit' and work began with some of that unit's clients. The two units opened simultaneously, preceded by two months of intensive staff training.

The Crisis Intervention Unit (CIU) is based on the ground floor. Like the long-stay unit, it also has room for ten residents at any one time. These can be individuals, couples, families (even people's domestic pets, or whatever social or domestic groups seem to need admission together at any time). There are facilities for people with babies, and children, and for people with physical handicaps. The unit is staffed by twelve mental health workers led by a team leader, all of whom are experienced in working in mental health emergency settings and have a wide variety of skills including welfare rights, individual and family counselling, relaxation skills and experience with problems relating to addictions to alcohol and drugs.

The unit operates 24 hours a day throughout the year and aims to respond quickly (within two hours) to requests for help. The staff work a shift system which ensures two or three workers on duty at all times, supported by the officer in charge or the team leader on duty at the unit or on call via a long distance 'bleep'. The unit defines a crisis as a situation in which one or more people are upset, sometimes by an obvious precipitator, and no longer feel they can cope by their usual methods.[2]

The unit works in a very simple, time-limited, goal-orientated way, over a maximum time limit of a month, to try to understand with people what has happened and why. We and they try to identify what has precipitated the 'upset', how to modify the effects, make sense of and deal with the present consequences and if possible prevent such an upset recurring. The minimum aimed for is a return of the client to 'previous coping levels'.[3] Clients can come into residence if that seems best; otherwise we work with people in the community, either visiting them in their homes or being visited by them at the centre. Telephone support is available at all times. The CIU takes referrals from anyone in the London Borough of Greenwich including self referrals. We will try to be helpful in any referred situation but do not usually deal directly with situations in which the main stated problem is alcohol or drug related, housing, or in which the person referred is under 17. The 'identified client' must also be willing for us to intervene, and be physically and mentally well enough to benefit even minimally from such intervention.

If the referral is from another professional agency we ask that the referrer jointly assess the situation with us. In the case of a self referral with no other agencies presently involved, workers from the CIU will assess the situation with the client. This enables consultation during assessment, between workers, and workers and the unit if there is access to a telephone. Most assessments take place at the referrer's point of contact. This gives mutual support to workers and also a wider information base for assessment. A 'key-worker' and 'co-worker' system is used; these workers in consultation with the team leader and officer in charge have prime responsibility to work out with their clients the best way to proceed, and leave detailed instructions for colleagues for work to be done in their absence if necessary. This way of working requires trust, co-operation and tolerance from all concerned, including clients, and has worked quite well so far.

In the first six months of operation the CIU received 235 referrals, made 71 assessments and admitted 34 people to residence at the unit. Formal counselling sessions with clients numbered 421, and 586 supportive telephone calls were made to clients. CIU made 347 support and advice/information calls to other agencies. The total number of agency contact calls – getting/giving information and advice on behalf of the CIU and its clients – was 2,026.

Analysis of the referrals shows the average age of CIU clients to be 35 years. Of those referred, 143 were women and 92 men. Self and family/friends referred 95, social service department workers 93, the health services 42 and virtually none from all other services.

Work continues in analysing the reasons why people contact the CIU. Indicators are that many crises are as a result of difficulties in life transitions: children leaving home, old age, new babies. Others are situational: loss of job, break-up of relationships, difficulties in the case of some clients from ethnic minorities of managing two cultures' expectations. Some present 'acute psychiatric emergencies' – overdoses, self harm through cutting, and harm from others by being physically, including sexually, abused. Some cases present initially as an 'identified client' showing 'psychotic features'. At present there seems to be no predictable pattern to referrals by a defined problem. Research based in the unit and outside it will eventually give some indication on such patterns of use. Some components of the referred's situations seem quite consistent. These are initial feelings by the referrer of confusion and uncertainty and a wish to act swiftly to get rid of these uncomfortable states.

The resolution of some aspects of referred problems has been achieved. These include housing and other welfare rights matters, the arrangement of physical health checks and basic home support systems. The satisfactory outcome of returning the 'identified client' and their social system to 'previous coping levels' is more difficult to evaluate and is less apparently helpful when those levels seem often to be quite unsatisfactory to all concerned. However people seem to benefit from the temporary asylum offered and the chance to rest. This recuperation from stress also seems valued by social workers whose clients are temporarily resident at the CIU.

Satisfactory onward referrals to long-term therapeutic support are difficult to make given a general lack of such support, and the wish by many of our clients and their professional and family carers to have a long-term difficulty resolved *now*. *All* of these difficulties will doubtless increase when we publicize the CIU work more widely in the near future.

Why then did Greenwich Council, operating in a climate of severe economic stringency (the borough is 'rate-capped'), feel it necessary to set up a unit, solely financed, managed and staffed by its social service department, specifically to practise mental health crisis intervention? How has this new service been received by professional and voluntary agencies in the locality? How have the CIU team and users dealt with being participants in this venture?

The answers to these questions circle around the concepts of glory, territory and power. As has been previously stated, Greenwich Council was faced with the reduction of material resources to deal with mental health problems perceived by its electorate and prominent council members to be in need of urgent expansion. Both these factors were seen in the borough to be a result of national government planning and re-organization. By 1984 the council, now predominantly left wing Labour, needed to agree the extensive and long overdue funding for the Lansdowne Lane Centre. This coincided with national government passing measures which drastically reduced the overall finance available to local authorities in the foreseeable future. In the face of such perceived corporate oppression the council flaunted its continued commitment to those people whom it saw as particularly powerless to resist the destructive forces imposed on them by national government edicts. The chance to make glorious – 'transform into something more splendid'[4] – that which otherwise presaged defeat did not pass the council and its leaders by. The fact that a neighbouring borough already boasted a similar project may also have encouraged their decision!

That the council chose to demonstrate its power in this way had considerable impact on the borough's other major social care agency, the district health authority. Its practitioners now found their ideology and practice directly confronted in the area of mental health. The council's own social services department whilst backing the venture overall also found some of its practitioners and managers angrily questioning why scarce resources had been used in this way. Health and social service personnel reaction to the setting up of the CIU often seemed to be expressed as versions of 'who do you think you are?' and/or 'give me some of that!' Such varying mixtures of contempt and envy may perhaps be seen in terms of a perceived attack on professional power, territory, and identity. In times of ever reducing resources, control over what one thinks one has become is increasingly urgent.

In dealing exclusively with mental distress crises the CIU places itself squarely in the operational area previously only dealt with in Greenwich by the health service. The CIU team refuses to see these crisis states in a solely 'medical model'. The team also makes a point of using everyday language, rather than that of medicine and especially psychiatry, to talk about how clients feel about and respond to situations. The CIU's use of specific goal-oriented, time-structured techniques to bring about rapid reduction of crisis situations, together with the standard use of written contracts of agreed action between referrers, CIU workers and clients, constitutes further a climate of an effective, different technology. That all participants agree equally in the written contract flattens the previous hierarchy of power in such situations. It is no longer the doctor who primarily defines the situation by naming the illness and ordering its treatment. The clients' power to name the situation – 'diagnosis' – and to participate in deciding how the situation should best be helped – 'treatment' – is now overtly acknowledged. Responsibility to effect the planned change is now more shared between the client and the care team.

This use of specific techniques and equipment, the initially narrowly limited area of focused questioning to identify the real nature of the presented problem, the often dramatic and speedy changes in behaviour that CIU intervention brings, place the CIU worker in the virtuoso role. Such a role within the field of mental health, incorporating apparently mysterious skills, understanding and effects, has until recently remained exclusively the property of psychiatrists. Its use by others, together with the secularization of the language which describes mental distress, questions the exclusive power and skill of the medical and psychiatric profession to understand and help in these crises.[5] 'A change of language can transform our appreciation of the Cosmos'.[6] Difficulties can arise for all participants when that appreciation involves alteration in previous assured levels of power and responsibility.

Not least are those difficulties a client faces when given the responsibility to identify and face for themselves the real nature of their problem and then do something about it. For some it quickly becomes preferable to retreat to the world of institutionalized psychiatry where others will decide what 'the problem' is and set about 'curing' you. Where the CIU observes this happening with clients they point it out to all participants in the system and whilst agreeing that change is often terrifying and difficult, the CIU will remove itself from involvement until the client chooses to be 'sane' rather than 'mad'.

Working within the overall structure of a large local authority social services department the work of the CIU again merges boundaries, works in other sectors' territories, uses its language to rename people's perceptions and responses. Because it has both residential and community facilities and works with both, primarily as CIU and client decide, it has an immediate access to and power over its resources that other colleagues in the department do not. It is up to the collective decision of the team on duty to decide in what way they will respond to a referral. The teams make these decisions as a routine part of their duty at any time of the day or night. They do not need to ratify their decisions with anyone else in the department. In practice, decisions are usually made with extensive consultation between involved colleagues in all disciplines but finally the allocation of resources of time, space and intensive therapeutic input are made by the team on duty. This freedom to immediately and actively allocate scarce resources is not available to other colleagues at practitioner level in the department.

Differences of opinion between colleagues in the department and the CIU as to 'the right way to proceed' occur on occasion. What is presented as a 'client crisis' may sometimes be renamed as a 'worker crisis' and the intervention be directed towards re-evaluating their position and supporting new and perhaps difficult decisions that may need to be made. Usually this interpretation of events is welcomed: at other times the referrer is irritated at having their formulation of 'the problem' rearranged and stalks off – 'I'll let you know if you're going to be needed.' All referrals, however apparently inappropriate, are responded to by a CIU team member and information, advice and active listening are given for all requests for support. A call-back system ensures that team members systematically check back to every referral within a week of initial contact to ask how things are now and if any further assistance is required. This part of the service seems particularly appreciated by colleagues.

However difficult and unsettling colleagues in health and social service settings have found the creation of the CIU, it must be said that overall the level of co-operation and appropriate interagency work is remarkably high and generally agreed by all participants to be so.

The CIU staff are employed by the social services department as residential social workers. As such they receive salaries that reflect the overall national lower pay to residential social workers when compared to field social workers. CIU staff necessarily practise both residential and field social work skills. They do not have any formal statutory responsibility in their practice but deal routinely with a wide range of field social work problems: these include child abuse, child sexual abuse, housing and welfare rights work, involvement with the work of the police, probation service and courts, and work concerned with aspects of fostering and adoption.

The CIU staff come from and have a wide range of backgrounds and professional qualifications. They are mostly quite young – under 30 – and relatively inexperienced in terms of years spent in practice settings.

To manage the CIU's difficult and stressful workload requires the staff to have humour, energy, creativity and the ability to think clearly and systematically in chaotic situations. This latter need is supported by the staff's initial professional training often in branches of psychiatric nursing or social work, and by the quite firm structures of evaluation and operation that the CIU uses. The whole team also participated in a week-long assertiveness training before the CIU opened designed specifically to help them present firmly and consistently their understanding of and response to a situation. Energy and creativity occasionally waver in the face of overwork due to staff absence or sickness: a flight into 'previous methods of coping' – diagnosis, labelling, the frantic search for the right book with *the answer*, have been noted. However, individually and collectively, interest and enthusiasm are high, and helpful responses to the work identified have been made.

The degree of autonomy that the CIU has over its working environment gives its workers a high level of responsibility. The stresses of this together with those of constantly dealing with very upset people and of horrifying circumstances are considerable. Support for individuals within the team and the CIU team overall is very necessary: regular individual and group supervision by the officer in charge and the team leader is a practised priority. The centre has allocated money from its revenue budget for weekly sessions with a consultant psychiatrist who advises on both client and team based concerns. She also provides an invaluable informal link with the hierarchy of the local medical and psychiatric systems.

The centre as a whole is also supported by consultation with the principal officer controlling the social services department's resident and day care resources. Last and by no means least, the CIU is very fortunate to work in a department whose director is a committed believer in the value of crisis intervention techniques.

The interlinking of political, economic and social factors often over decades provides major factors in both causation of and response to mental health problems. Crises can usually be seen coming from afar, on a national, family or individual level. The response often seems one of wholesale 'closure' against 'the problem' (often presented as being in 'the problem's' best interests of course!): close hospitals, move towards community care (without sufficient resources for the community to do so), put the identified client in hospital, take them away *now*. In the end it doesn't work and people become by turns angry and despairing. What does seem to alleviate crises is a willingness to listen to what people say they want and try to provide as much of that as possible as soon as possible, even if it is only on a very basic level. Economic, social and personal limitations on such provision should be explained carefully and if necessary firmly. Personal responsibility to improve these limitations should be encouraged and supported.

Greenwich Social Services Department's response to mental health crises in the borough has been an attempt to do these things. The Lansdowne Lane Centre is one part of an expanding mental health service which is planning further residential and community-based support in consultation with service providers and consumers. The spirit of the Unicorn – hope and imagination in the face of difficulty – is alive and well.

Disclaimer
The London Borough of Greenwich accepts no responsibility for the author's opinions or conclusions contained in this chapter.

References

1. Ratna, L. (1978) *The Practice of Psychiatric Crisis Intervention*, Napsbury Hospital League of Friends, St. Albans.
2. Caplan, G. (1974) *Principles of Preventative Psychiatry*, Basic Books Inc., New York.
3. Ibid.
4. *The Concise Oxford Dictionary* (1974) 5th edition, Oxford University Press, p. 522.
5. Huntingdon, J. (1981) *Social Work and General Medical Practice: Collaboration or Conflict?*, George Allen & Unwin, London, p. 83.
6. Lee Whorf, B. (1965) *Language, Thought and Reality: Selected writing of,* J.B. Carron (ed), MIT Press, Cambridge, Massachusetts, p. vii.

4

Approaching Mental Distress

GIUSEPPE DELL'ACQUA, ROBERTO MEZZINA

Crisis and the Psychiatric Circuit

The Persistence of the Psychiatric Hospital, the Medical Model and Simplification

It is difficult to give an unambiguous definition of crisis in psychiatry. Whatever the frame of reference, any definition must ultimately take account of the existing psychiatric organization in that area at a specific point in time.

A person in crisis is likely to enter the psychiatric system in which the psychiatric hospital is the last resort.

The 'threshold value' of entry into the psychiatric circuit will be redefined from time to time according to the recognition of thresholds, such as those of suffering, social disorder, social danger, poverty, the weight given to the family, social or work relationships, diversity of behaviour, intolerance or violence in that particular social network.

In various countries crisis intervention centres often use quick, early methods of treatment aimed at solving the problem as soon as possible outside the psychiatric circuit. In particular they try to reduce the number of hospital admissions.

We believe, however, that these therapeutic interventions are short-term and do not make use of methods which offer overall care to the patient in crisis. Consequently they cannot provide for the eventuality of failure and often have recourse to 'heavier' institutions which lead finally to the psychiatric hospital. In this way the centrality of the psychiatric hospital is sustained.

The psychiatric circuit, assured of the psychiatric hospital, has developed into a highly complex, specialist working model. But its model of cultural reference has not changed at all. All the practices developed by it continue to use separate lines of intervention and to fragment the response to a person's needs into various therapies.

Any course of therapy with an infinite number of options is usually difficult to negotiate for those who really need it. Paradoxically, the choice of highly diversified services is often disproportionate to the opportunities available for using them. Further, the inflexibility in access, in referral and in the other phases of the circuit not only fail to resolve a crisis but often provoke one.

Because the system cannot recognize the patient as a complex entity, it is simplistic and reductive. It is always the patient's crisis which is seen, never the crisis of a system which cannot cope with an overwhelming number of requirements.

The moment when a person in crisis is given attention can be identified as the point of greatest simplification. The individual has already gradually reduced the complexity of his suffering to symptoms so that they might be noticed. The service responds by equipping itself to perceive only those symptoms.

Integrated District Service: the Case for Complexity
In this work we intend to record our experience in Trieste and to try to show how conditions of crisis actually correspond to very complex life situations and how resources and methods aimed at protecting such situations should be complex too.

In fact, the concept of crisis in psychiatry arises out of an intention, correct at a theoretical level, to reassess mental illness by investigating suffering in the individual's life. The individual must be viewed as a 'biological unit' as well as a 'member of a microsocial system' and even as a 'social individual'.

In this sense the concept of crisis has been an attempt to apply a single methodology. It does not produce uniformity but specifically seeks out the individual nature of the problems presented by the user. By examining the patient's individual history the symptom too can be identified as a significant factor, part of a reality which has now become intelligible.

In our experience the many occasions for contact between the service and the individual (in the places where s/he lives, has a network of relationships, and material problems) can be used to reconstruct a person's life history. This helps to locate the crisis within a series of relationships which in turn render it comprehensible (but do not explain it!). Finally, it helps to salvage the valuable connection between health, life values and the crisis.

In our case, the phasing out of psychiatric hospitals in the 1970s and the establishment of mental health centres – the final phase of de-institutionalization – has created a practical and conceptual problem. It is the problem of understanding complexity which exists wherever there is a demand for psychiatry and wherever there is a crisis.

The specific mental health centre (MHC) in which we work operates in a small district. It is equipped to deal with all requests which elsewhere would be identified as psychiatric, and to eliminate any administrative filters. It favours means of access which are informal and varied. It does not attempt either to select or to refer patients elsewhere.

The mental health service therefore assumes a central position within the defined area. It becomes a totally unique point of observation, in which interactive observation can be developed. It will reflect everything which the population may produce in terms of pathology, deprivation, conflict and social disorder; it will be protracted constantly and steadily over time; it will follow personal histories and the evolution of that district and its population. The service will therefore be able to adapt its response accordingly.

The service is capable of identifying and entering into contact with and working out the conflictual network of relationships which constitute a crisis. These might otherwise have been hidden, trivialized or made devoid of meaning by the process of simplification which usually takes place wherever the working model is based on the centrality of the psychiatric hospital.

The most difficult problem is the need for an organizational model of the service which will encourage appropriate responses to complex individual situations as and when they emerge.

The Work of the Mental Health Centre

Contact

The way in which acute patients come into contact with the psychiatric circuit in Trieste has been significantly altered as a result of the 15 years of work. Once the only means of access was by compulsory admission to the psychiatric hospital, which was finally closed in 1980. By 1985, 75 per cent of all crisis situations were referred directly to the MHC. Thus the public and the network of public services have become aware of the district service and are able to use it.

Increasingly it is the workers at the centre who are called upon in the first instance when a request for treatment is made. Contact with the patient at the first signs of crisis can differ in time and mode. If the patient does not present himself at the centre, the workers soon take an active role in establishing contact. Wherever possible the places of contact will be those where the patient spends his time naturally (the home, the bar, the workplace, etc.) and the means will be significant people in his environment. The service is prepared to be as flexible as possible in this regard. It does not operate according to predetermined records of treatment nor with specialist teams.

More often than not, actually being 'on the spot' prevents traumatic incidents: the worker's presence in itself gives immediate reassurance to relatives and neighbours. It can defuse a crisis which is causing anguish to the patient and to whoever is closest to him. Sometimes, however, it is not possible to defuse a situation, usually in cases where the patient is alone, with few resources and few relationships with the outside world. Such a person will obstinately refuse contact and isolate himself still further. The service then has to increase its 'low-key' approach: telephone calls, messages under the door, involving others such as friends, the priest, the local policeman or the plumber; or even attempts to make contact in several places. These attempts give determined proof of attention and help and in this way the service tries to engage in a reciprocal relationship.

At other times, a sort of escalation is identified and continued refusal induces the service to pay greater attention to the user's informal, yet contractual, power and to his requests: thus the service is increasingly obliged to show its flexibility. In the end the escalation can conclude with physical contact with the patient which can be both dramatic and strong. Opening the closed door (rarely with police co-operation) is a symbol for the breaking of the psychotic circle, for the entrance of real faces and for the end of a nightmare.

In short, the stress of so many tensions removes even the most obstinate barricade. Even when the patient persists in seeing the service or the worker as an intruder, those moments of offering, listening and practical help (both in the home and in the centre) manage to break down any diffidence and to create a worker-patient relationship. The therapy programme can be started.

Treatment and Liberation

The service must be able to recognize the signs of an unexpressed crisis which cannot be heard. Such a crisis could lead to alarming behaviour as a sign of suffering, and eventually social emergency systems may be activated.

The service must also be able to organize different types of contact. In this way any crisis will be placed within a single practice for prevention, cure and rehabilitation. In fact response to crisis cannot be detached from secondary preventive work since this is correctly based on the practice of taking overall responsibility for the factors in question.

We would argue that waiting for the client on the service premises and laying down rigid rules for treatment leads to the traumatic mechanics of compulsory treatment or to the intervention of the police and, for acute cases, subsequent hospitalization in wards.

Concerning the demand for social control (which is always connected to the demand for treatment), the CMHC's existence will redefine a mental patient's much-feared dangerousness and allow him an alternative means of expression. It will also mean that this expression, with the help of the service, will be understood by those s/he mixes with.

It has become clear that conflict, including crisis, means a conflict of power in which the user – in so far as s/he is identified as such – experiences a net loss. This happens even when s/he appears to retain the manipulative dominance exercised by the symptoms. In any case conflict occurs within a predicament which immobilizes the user and others around him and from which nobody can escape.

If one of the aims of the service is to seek out all avenues of freedom for users, it shall equip itself, as in our case, with methods and resources designed to encourage growth and autonomy. This will then depend on and increase the contractual nature of the relationship between the client and the service. Supporting the client's power and autonomy in this way does not mean calling upon sterile guarantees for defending patients' rights as individuals. It is based instead on a programme of change for all concerned, including psychiatric workers.

Assuming Full Responsibility

Taking responsibility refers primarily to the service's *active responsibility* for the mental health of the whole of its area. The service becomes an active agent for 'social control', a function inherited from the old mental hospital system. However, this function must be restyled when operating at district level. Workers who are directly present must relinquish traditional systems of control. They must reduce to a minimum any delay between the time when a problem emerges and the time when contact is made. This practice strengthens the link between the service and the district, makes it more direct and facilitates conditions for reciprocal relationships.

The user's social context is not bureaucratically separated out into various areas of functioning. The individual is accompanied, or supported, by the service throughout the network of social institutions (court, prison, hospital, welfare office, school, youth services, housing department, family meetings, rest homes, benefit offices, etc.) which have been activated by the service in response to the user's needs.

Taking responsibility means overcoming in a practical way the opposite of the institutionalized out-patient's clinic, a typical product of the medical model.

Taking responsibility does not mean that a specific setting for it must be established. The place for intervention can be the mental health centre, or other social institutions (the general hospital, the prison, etc.). Preferably it should be in the user's environment, where s/he tries to live his social life.

Even when treatment for the crisis takes place in the mental health centre by the various means of hospitality which are open 24 hours a day, users continue the relationship with their environment. Relatives and friends can visit at any time. Often the client will be accompanied back home soon after times of great stress in order to collect clothes and personal belongings, to see relatives and to check the conditions and existence of a home with a worker. All this is designed to guarantee and communicate to the person that the arrival at the centre does not mean breaking with life's continuity. The client may also go outside the centre, alone or accompanied by a worker, volunteer, relative or another patient, so that s/he can see that s/he has not lost his/her own autonomy or freedom.

In this way, space in the centre acquires symbolic connotations as a place for relationships and as a wider therapeutic community. It does not become a place where the person is limited or temporarily segregated. Confidential relationships are designed to rebuild the user's identity and/or repair relationships which had broken down before the crisis (including by hospitalization).

Sometimes a user will leave the centre, renewing the refusal and breaking the relationship of trust and friendship which has been established. In this event the workers are obliged to find them, re-establish contact, and review their demands at the new contractual level suggested by breaking the relationship. The flexible management structure, as well as the ways of taking responsibility described above, does not mean that the service fails to recognize the need to protect individuals who behave alarmingly and who risk being exposed to sanctions from instruments of social control (for example, an ordinary or psychiatric prison).

In all of these situations the centre assumes responsibility for keeping control and providing safeguards for patients, but it never uses physical means of restraint or closed doors. This includes bans on leaving the centre, limitations on movement or on contact with relatives and pharmacological sedation. But the work is personalized by the figure of the worker who follows, assists and 'accompanies' the patient continually. S/he also gives explanations to and motivates the patient by trying to create a greater awareness.

Hospitality at the centre forms part of a series of gestures and events which precede, accompany and follow it. It is always part of a course of treatment and never a response to crisis in itself. By concentrating on the way hospitality is managed within the service, more human energy and institutional resources can be brought into play so that the attention of the whole centre can be focused on the client.

The experience of hospitality at the centre for ourselves and both direct users and their relatives is that the practical and symbolic dismantling operation takes the form of 'asylum' proper. Because the institution's operation is very open, changes in demand can be identified and responded to. In our experience the demand for total segregation and internment no longer exists.

The Therapeutic Programme

Organized Listening

When a patient in crisis arrives at the centre, s/he is never subjected to a psychiatric consultation which, using professional knowledge, is aimed solely at diagnosing and objectivizing him/her. Usually an attempt is made to establish a relationship in which each party gradually gets to know the other and in which several workers and sometimes other users are involved. The new person is given time to adjust to the space in the centre.

An atmosphere where people are readily available encourages many exchanges and interactions between users, professionals and other members of staff (for example cooks, cleaners, linen-keepers and co-operative users trained for this type of work), other patients and voluntary workers. Often collective discussions and meetings take place spontaneously and these are encouraged by the professionals. Several clients can be involved in these and in it they would have to face each other as they come to know the problems and communication levels of other people.

Even the daily lunchtime meetings in which professionals communicate information and thoughts, do not exclude users. In fact, they are encouraged to participate and they either listen to or comment on the topics being discussed. Sometimes a client is inspired to speak out about what s/he considers to be his/her 'own problem'. On these occasions, they are listened to and given collective recognition. The 'problem' comes to the attention of the group without there being any attempt to interpret it. These 'informal' moments are often the most important and useful to clients in crisis situations.

Formalized occasions for listening – that is, a defined space and time for conversation between professionals and an individual user – are never laid down for a psychotherapy which follows predetermined models. They are inserted into and are part of the varied occasions when people listen and get to know one another. Usually, conversation is designed to make it easier for the person to express the needs which underlie the request for psychiatric treatment, and to encourage comparison between the person's real-life situation and contradictions regarding his/her current condition. It is designed to analyse what happened when the illness began, to relate the condition to the personal life history and to connect it with real life by examining and sharing her/his life and social experiences before the illness. This reconstruction reduces the user's anxiety. It is then possible to identify the current problems to be dealt with and draw up a practical programme. The programme will take account of the user's capabilities, how to increase them, and of the resources which the service can offer itself or try to make available elsewhere.

Both formal occasions for listening and the more numerous informal occasions seem to make people aware of being with others, of listening to their own and other people's needs, of restraining themselves and limiting their self-centredness. It will be evident that all this does not happen naturally but needs to be supported by well-defined work, with clear objectives, by a highly skilled team.

The Use of Time, or the Art of Relating

When hospitalized, patients live totally inside the time and pace of the institution which contains them. Thus time, which co-ordinates our experiences, is taken away from them. Hospitalization separates 'ill time' from 'normal and healthy time', spanning through the crisis.

The time lived by a person in crisis can, however, be expressed in an autonomous form in the MHC, turning it into a fundamental tactical factor in the intervention process. The time passed in contact with the service can become filled with acts, presence and presentations useful for a person in crisis, such as discussing with him/her his proposals and initiatives and demonstrating respect for the decisions how to use one's own time.

Inside such a centre a primary network of relationships evolves around the users: relationships of involvement, affection and mutual support. Though born inside the centre these are often carried over to the outside world too, especially within the users' group. Thus new forms of conviviality, economic support, tolerance and solidarity are developed.

This complexity can encourage the multiplicity of expressions and behaviours which in turn enables individuals to find their own space. In the centre we observe the coexistence of people with acute and chronic problems, old and young, different levels of pathology and social class. This fact demonstrates not only that such a mixture is possible, but also its usefulness in confronting the variety of personalities, the fear of madness and in facilitating the development of understanding of other people's problems. For the workers, this complexity enables them to have a wide view and to prevent sterile specialisms. It leads to a focus on variety of practices too.

Outside the centre, the different workshops which exist in Trieste (for example, theatre, painting, sailing) enrich the network of the services by offering another path in which the ability to relate can be reconstructed. In the non-specific, yet diverse, contexts of the centre the possibility of sharing the experience facilitates the expression, containment and the recompensation of the crisis.

The Therapeutic Offer: the Social Reproduction in the Crisis

The first contacts between the centre and the user focus on finding out what are the latter's basic needs in their social and historical context; where does he live, sleep, what does he eat, how much is spent on drinking, etc. This marks the beginning of the therapeutic offer.

Practical support is offered as a natural progression, including all spheres of everyday life (for example, financial benefits, home help, lunch at the centre, leisure activities). Accompanying the user to a variety of places forms an integral part of the daily work. These maintain and activate the user's contact with the external environment as well as the informal relationships with the centre. This practice seems to reduce the time taken to respond to a particular need. It can also adapt itself better to the urgent demands placed upon it by users in crisis and thus contributes to resolving the crisis itself.

Responding to need implies providing first of all material means for social reproduction and for improving the quality of life. Then, gradually, profound and continuous change in the operation and philosophy of the service can take place. It increases the contractual nature of the user-service relationship and repositions the client within his/her context. The therapeutic results of this treatment have been witnessed by us even though they are often dismissively interpreted as 'welfare/comforting'. Work which has been developed around crisis as a response to need is therapeutic because it continually offers different workers real opportunities of relating to clients. It allows technical language to be immediately translated into the language of practical problems. This prevents the tendency in psychiatry to dismiss anything to do with the material nature of everyday life as irrelevant. It promotes practical exchange between the various individuals concerned and encourages the practice of accompanying clients.

We do not pretend to effect a change of the needs which underlie the psychiatric issue, but to provide responses which reinforce the process of the reacquisition of social identity and contractual power.

The Crisis of the Service: Breaking Down and Reconstructing the Institutional Equilibrium

The work with users can neither be carried out nor be understood properly without the complementary part of working on the nature of the service. The personalized therapeutic programme described above materializes within the conflict between the organization of the service and the specific problems posed by the users. A high degree of flexibility is required, which becomes possible only if a collective style of work is adopted. The style is expressed in the daily staff meetings, the constant exchange among the workers, and between workers and clients. Space for autonomous work for the different disciplines was created in the process of de-institutionalization. Likewise the hierarchical structure was reduced considerably in favour of a more horizontal division of labour.

This mode of work is not a given, but a possibility which requires constant effort to be maintained: the service is an institutional space and as such continuously reproduces regressive aspects of institutionalization, either in the users' relations with the service, or in the way the workers relate to their work.

It is always possible to come across the distance between worker and patient, the lack of attention, the objectivization, the breach of trust, the passive induction of chronicity. The capacity of a service to meet the challenge posed by problems, to live them as a 'proper' crisis, implies a non-linear progression, often through seemingly 'disordered' processes, at a cost of conflicts and the risk of becoming 'burnt out' and the reproduction of institutional life. Thus the emergence of the capacity to respond anew to the crisis is the outcome of the daily hard work on the modification of the neo-institutionalized mechanisms in the functioning of the service.

The organizational system needs to stay in a constant 'imbalance'. This is created by the different, and often contradictory, instances of work; by the different professional figures, always in a quarrel over the corporative defence of their professionality, the conflict between the satisfaction of the subjective needs and the wider response to the needs of the service. These are also the issues which require the development of an overall strategy. The complexity is helped by the richness of practice knowledge and the similarity between grassroots workers and the users in class and language.

The inherent contradictions in the work of the service are eased by creating the right relationships between identification with the users and distancing the affective and anxiety load of the collective, thus achieving a balance between individual investment and group support. In this sense – as well as in others – the centre is an enlarged therapeutic community, which acts both inside and outside its own life and space.

Conclusion

Instead of indicating a private solution to users' problems, we have attempted to arrive at a rapid normalization of the person. As usual in the strategies of 'crisis intervention' the responses to the crisis of the centre require to be interrelated, to put the user in contact with a system of relations, with human and material resources. Once this takes place, the crisis evolves in a collective environment. Provided the user goes through the crisis while maintaining his existential and historical continuity, the crisis loses its fragmented character and instead assumes a dynamic value. In our experience the event/illness tends to be transformed profoundly, either in its modality of expression or in its solution during the process of work in the centre.

The service cannot have the suppression of the symptoms as an objective, or be limited by an artificial end of the therapy for bureaucratic and technocratic reasons. As the centre wishes essentially to offer the means of social reproduction to the person in crisis, a brief duration of the support is not an aim in itself. Obviously, the possibility remains that the therapeutic programme might fail, due either to the limitations of the service or to the persistence of the illness as a personal and social sign to be decoded. In all, for a service like ours, the failure is both the outcome and the motivation for daily work because it determines the rethinking of the intervention.

The choice of the specific type of therapeutic relationships outlined above, intended as our temporary taking-on of full responsibility, does not follow the concept of recovery in the clinical sense, since for us the issue is to ensure the continuity of the user's life in the community. The real objective from our perspective is achieved when the person takes control over his/her life. The service is less preoccupied with the risk of the client becoming dependent, because it focuses on long-term transformations in which the user may mature to new levels of needs and the possibilities of expressing them.

References

For further reading on the centre's work, see:

1. Cogliati, M.G., Dell'Acqua, G. (1982) 'La banale quotidianità del C.S.M. di Barcola', *Fra regole e utopia* (ed) Cooperativa Psichiatria Democratica.

2. Cogliati, M.G., Dell'Acqua, G., Mezzina, R. (1984) 'I Servizi Psichiatri ci Forti tra Pericolosità, Perizia, Carcere, Manicomio Giudiziara', *Atti del Convegno, Capacità di intende re e di volere, Diritto e Psichiatria dopo la legge 180*, 1978, Università di Trieste.

3. Dell'Acqua, G., Cogliati, M.G. (1984) 'The end of the mental hospital', *Acta Psy. Scand.*, suppl. nr. 316.

4. Dell'Acqua, G., Mezzina, R., et al. (1981) 'Il territorio fra sanità e assistenza, Convegno Nazionale di Psichiatria Democratica', in *Fogli d'Informazione* 75–6.

5. Dell'Acqua, G., Mezzina, R., (1981) 'Per una critica della crisi', *Atti del Convegno, La crisi in psichiatria: Modelli interpretativi ed operativi*, Provincia di Milano.

6. Gaglio, A., Mezzina, R. (1983) 'Sul circuito psichiatrico triestino', *Fogli d'Informazione* 93–4.

5

Dependency or Autonomy

STEEN MANGEN

> As a committee, we have found it difficult in hearing the authentic voice of the ultimate consumer of community care ... Services are still mainly designed by providers and not users.
> Second Report of the Social Services Committee (Short Report), 1985[1]

The Short Report hardly makes reassuring reading about the progress made so far in the reformulation of health and social services in Britain. Yet, their indictment of current practice will not surprise critics of the organization-focused planning procedures characteristic of the British welfare state. Planners in the NHS, for example, have been primarily concerned with attempts to find an efficient and equitable means of allocating scarce health resources across regions and specialities. The result has been a system that has given professionals, and especially doctors, great gatekeeping powers, justified on the grounds that in many cases patients do not know what is good for them. Thus, once patients take the decision to consult – and in the case of psychiatry this decision is sometimes taken over their heads – they have generally had little active role in treatment plans being made by professionals on their behalf.

In recent years, however, there have been signs of an attempt to take the recipients of health and social services more seriously. In this chapter I will examine how this new role of 'patient-as-consumer', by promoting the individual's sense of autonomy, can contribute to better service management and the planning of new provisions. I will largely be concerned with a clientele receiving long-term day care. Many of these clients have previously been in-patients and are typical in certain respects of the chronic in-patient population to be discharged from psychiatric hospitals in coming years, in line with government plans to shed one third of the current bed capacity in England. Finally, I will review some relevant literature and also introduce some recent studies carried out in Camberwell, London, in which I have participated.

The Limits of Autonomy

Attempts to integrate patients in the planning process form part of the endeavours to reorientate mental health care more explicitly towards the restitution of an abiding sense of autonomy in individuals who, for a number of reasons, have become a highly dependent group. As an absolute, personal autonomy is the freedom to act and choose between options according to one's own priorities. In reality, of course, it is a relative concept, its parameters being determined by the interaction of a range of psychological, social, economic and political variables. The attempt to maintain autonomy involves a dynamic struggle to reconcile conflicts between the demands of personal and social identity. It is the irreconcilability of these conflicts which, for some groups, contributes to their social marginalization. Thus efforts to promote greater autonomy among the mentally ill are closely linked to theories of normalization (i.e. the development of culturally-valued role-playing) and psychiatric rehabilitation must be judged in terms of the degree to which agency is restored to clients in a measure consonant with their personal attributes, long-term disabilities and life situations.

Rehabilitation programmes frequently rely on a surrogate indicator of personal autonomy which is equated with the client's ability to plan and perform everyday activities independently. Where this is deficient remedial action at the individual level is required to limit the impact of psychological, social and economic constraints on the person's psychosocial performance. Specific interventions aimed at reducing the disabling effects of long-standing symptoms and institutional living are a prerequisite for the success of such programmes, so that through rehabilitation the client may learn positive skills of assertiveness in which the exercise of self-control, the essential basis of personal autonomy, gradually replaces reliance on externally imposed controls.

Beyond these immediate psychotherapeutic concerns, there are a range of problems about promoting autonomy among a socially deprived group which cannot be resolved within the confines of a service system. Directly at issue is the marginalized position of the long-term mentally ill in society, a status seriously reducing life chances, which they share with other 'at risk' groups managed by social welfare agencies. Their common social handicap stems from their denial of access to the full rights of citizenship which extend beyond conventional civil and political rights to rights to economic and social welfare.[2] Viewed from this perspective, many long-term users of psychiatric services are profoundly disadvantaged: their relative poverty imposes massive restrictions on choices available to them in daily life and, thus, can be the major determinant of the level of autonomy they attain. Most deprived are those patients with long histories of hospitalization, who are unlikely to have accumulated savings or other material possessions, so that their range of options on such matters as housing and leisure pursuits may be markedly restricted.

In attempting to overcome these far-reaching constraints, most British mental health workers have relied on traditional professional spheres of action, providing broadly-drawn occupational rehabilitation programmes. One effect of this preferred mode of operation has been to underplay any political implications of their interventions with clients, in sharp contrast to many of their Italian colleagues. The reasons are complex and have to do with the preservation of a 'neutral' professional ethos, as well as the continued fragmentation of much mental health training, so that collectively professionals do not speak with one voice. Equally important, of course, are the political views held by each agent, especially with regard to the degree to which s/he subscribes to strong redistributive goals in social policy.

Planning: An Authentic Voice for the Client?

One criterion of the success of promoting autonomy through developing consumerism is the degree to which users influence and are seen to influence the kinds of services delivered. In designing new provisions the need to engage the consumer at the earliest possible stage is all the more urgent because planning in large bureaucracies like the health and social services is inherently remote from the lives of the people they are ostensibly there to serve. All too often, existing types of services are merely reproduced, with the continued failure to mould provisions around the individual needs of the clients rather than the reverse. Yet, the mere consultation of clients in planning will not be enough for, contrary to the tendency in official reports, we cannot naively assume that a broad consensus exists among users and planners and that the integration of the client into the planning process will proceed unproblematically. The risk, then, of merely conferring a bogus participatory role on users is very real: their views may be accepted only when they support the preferences of providers and may be ignored when they do not easily conform to current administrative responsibilities. The practice of discharging long-stay patients to their original 'home' areas is a case in point. Patients' wishes have often been neglected, with the policy being dictated by the concern to distribute responsibilities for future care among sectorized social services.

Although the degree to which agency is restored to users in the planning of psychiatric provisions must naturally be appropriate to their individual attributes, the goal should always be to make services less coercive in operation and less stigmatizing and marginalizing in effect. Critics of the new community-based services created in Britain and elsewhere have deep reservations about the progress made so far in this direction. They complain of the continuance of hospital-centrism, in ideology if not in physical location, and of the excessive reliance on professionalization in creating a therapeutic milieu. The result, they claim, is that day care and residential services continue to foster dependency among many clients capable of exercising a greater degree of autonomy. Foucault,[3] for instance, believes that institutionalism has merely been transferred to the community, where it breeds in what he picturesquely – albeit melodramatically – maps out as a 'carceral archipelago' of day and out-patient services, workshops and residential units.

Foucault's provocative turn of phrase is unlikely to receive a favourable reception among many professionals trained in the Anglo-Saxon tradition who will regard it as a gross distortion of the positive effects of locally-based services created over the past 30 years. Yet, few of them would argue that the present community services are ideal in terms of organization and operational style, or would deny that at least the vestiges of institutionalism can be observed among some of their clientele. Several factors are implicated. One problem for day units who have tried to implement active rehabilitation is that many of their clients coming from the in-patient sector have received inadequate preparation whilst still in hospital, forcing them to provide instead long-term support and containment. The relative scarcity of day care provisions means that many units are required to accept too wide a range of clients, creating problems compounded by very low staff ratios. Overplacement and underplacement are therefore rife, with the risk of clients being allocated to rehabilitation programmes that are not catering for their specific needs.

Yet, criticisms of current practices in day services cannot be sufficiently explained solely in terms of the inappropriate allocation of clientele, limited provisions and low staff ratios. The research to be reviewed here indicates that the chosen style of operation of some day and residential units is not directed towards exploiting the potential for autonomy that their clients possess. It follows that the study of autonomy cannot be restricted to the patient alone, but must incorporate the interactive effects on users, professionals and service provisions. The patient may be confronted with the novel situation of having his views solicited when previously his role was merely to provide information to be used as clinical 'material'. Patient dependency carries its own rewards for professionals, so that, as Watts and Bennett[4] remark: 'caring about patients frequently reduces to caring for them.' Clinical staff will therefore have to accept that the promotion of autonomy requires them to be genuinely engaged in a renegotiation of long-established roles, the outcome of which must be the eradication of paternalistic attitudes and a reduction of social distance in clinical relationships that such dependency has sustained. It is likely that the feedback obtained in these new relations will not always support cherished professional practices or existing modes of service. Yet, the change of approach to clients is vital if we are to develop a more responsive network of services. However difficult the process, it must surely represent a considerable improvement on the present situation where often the only action patients feel able to take to register dissatisfaction with their treatment is through non-compliance, irrespective of whether or not this leads to positive outcomes. Wolfensberger[5] has examined these issues in greater detail in his work on normalization. His conclusions apply equally in this context and have fundamental implications, not only for approaches to planning, but also for the future training of mental health professionals: normalization is not merely something 'done' to a person, but is a principle for designing and delivering services.

Some Satisfaction Studies
Many studies have been small-scale and have involved highly articulate groups, portraying in some detail the quality of the patients' lives. Direct utility to planning has been a secondary consideration. It is clear from Brandon's review of British studies that the primary focus is the patient who has suffered from acute or episodic illnesses.[6] It is comparatively rare for the voice of the long-term patient to be heard.

Emerging from these studies is the general feeling among in-patients that, at best, they have a marginal say in critical decisions affecting their future, especially in the process of discharge 'to the community'. Most studies have underlined the blow to self-esteem that follows hospital admission. The situation cannot be helped by the poor flow of information about the illness, prognosis and medication from clinical staff to patients and their relatives; nor by the lack of privacy, lack of storage space for personal belongings and noise at night which disturbs sleep (for example, King's Fund Centre).[7] These intrusions on the person may lead to a rapid loss of motivation, a state which is directly related to length of stay.[8] Such results underline the need of engaging patients at all stages in the planning of their treatment programme so that skills and self-confidence can be built up, as well as feelings of mastery about decisions for the future. In practice, however, discharge is often thrust upon unsuspecting patients, who not unnaturally may be deeply anxious about their life outside. As if this were not bad enough, the imposition of an abrupt discharge often takes the form of an arbitrary solution: some patients report that they were led to believe there were no alternatives and felt that pressure was put on them to acquiesce quickly, with little time to think things over or to be able to change their minds. This unsatisfactory situation is exacerbated by the fact that information on sources of advice about such matters as housing and social security is either inadequate or non-existent.[9]

Patients outside hospital may fare no better. Although day care, for example, is often encountered as a positive experience and preferable to the in-patient ward, some patients complain of a rigid and boring programme with little variety or choice. Because of a lack of alternative facilities and the inability to express their consumer preferences owing to a very low income, some clients see the day unit as the only way of spending the day that provides them with a modicum of 'sheltered leisure'. Once there, they may feel they have to put up with other 'therapeutic programmes' in which they have no real interest but in which there may be heavy encouragement from staff to participate. Others may resent the imposition by some day units of compulsory daily attendance, especially where their hostel place is dependent on it.[10] It is not surprising, therefore, that it is day patients living in hostels who are the most likely to complain of a highly structured and institutionalized environment, in which they hover between the regulations of the hostel and those of the day unit.[11]

The continued lack of active social rehabilitation both inside and outside hospital is amply demonstrated by many studies. One serious deficiency in particular is the frequent absence of social skills training. Many former in-patients complain of the poverty of mutually rewarding social relationships outside hospital, so that life 'in the community' can be profoundly isolated, to the detriment of their self-esteem.[12] Yet, at the same time, these respondents may record their deep resentment of the degree of communality enforced on them in hostels and day units and are especially critical of being forced to share with room-mates they have not freely chosen.[13]

The Camberwell Studies

These studies have focused on samples of long-term day clientele attending NHS, local authority and voluntary sector provisions, many of whom also live in a variety of sheltered accommodation. An important conclusion of an earlier study in this series was that few of the local day services in the sample had been planned with the promotion of autonomy as a prime consideration, with the result that insufficient opportunities were given to individual clients to practise certain skills they already possessed.[14] Residential facilities were equally, if not more, at fault: for, surely, the image of a hostel as home is sorely tarnished if, as in the majority in this study, residents are required to inform the staff about their whereabouts at weekends, where staff may enter bedrooms without permission and where residents do not help plan meals and are not allowed to consume alcohol on the premises.[15]

A more recent study is concerned with day unit attenders' perceptions of their skills and with their expressed motivations to perform tasks. Particularly common were the deficits clients perceived in their ability to form and maintain social relationships. Equally important was the discovery that half the tasks specified by the researchers (for instance, household chores), which are typical components of social rehabilitation programmes in day units, were regarded as unimportant by the respondents.[16]

These observations have immediate implications for the organization of occupational and industrial therapy in day services. In fact, one of the day hospitals in our sample has recently initiated a procedure in which patients will be regularly asked about their attitudes to individual programmes on offer, irrespective of whether they are currently involved in them. The introduction of this monitoring system was prompted by the relatively low attendance at optional activities, suggesting that this day unit may not be allocating the right things to the right people. A substantial level of unmet demand has been uncovered in the new approach, with clear indications that clients want to be able at least to try activities they have never been offered. Most popular among these activities are baking, photography, music and learning how to use the microcomputer. It is hoped that the new system will provide a useful monitoring and feedback service so that occupational therapy can respond more swiftly to clients' needs, as well as giving clients a real role in shaping their daily programme.[17]

The aim of our study of long-term day care is to design a procedure for the regular assessment of the needs of the individual client which takes into account positive attributes, disabilities and life situations. Two measurements of need have been developed: 'need for care' – the need for specific interventions (for example, counselling) that could be provided by a variety of lay and professional agents; and 'need for services' – the identification of an appropriate setting for the delivery of service.

In order to make our assessments, we found that we had to solicit information from a large number of respondents: clients, relatives, various members of the clinical team and hostel and day centre staff. In many cases clients proved to be the most important informants about needs. However, they could only be one of the sources of response, for their report of problems could be incomplete. We identified needs of which the client had, at best, imperfect knowledge – need for medication review is such an instance. Yet, these situations apart, clients could not in any case have been the sole determiners of how their problems are translated into needs for some kind of formal intervention, since professionals must establish the legitimacy of the need and accord it some priority in the attempt to ensure that resources are rationed fairly and efficiently.

According to our criteria, just over half of the sample of 145 day unit attenders had problems in structuring their day or in managing their household affairs without direction; 45 per cent had deficits in managing money; and 45 per cent lacked sufficient skills in social interaction which restricted their ability to form relationships outside the shelter of the psychiatric services. These sorts of deficits had to be taken into account in assessing the degree to which currently the client could effectively act independently. The necessity of monitoring clients' needs is indicated by our observation that a substantial level of unmet need for individual elements of care can exist alongside quite high levels of overprovision, a situation that can foster dependency. Over half the sample had at least one unmet need which we judged serious enough to warrant action.[18] Equally important was the substantial amount of overplacement of clients in too dependent a setting. For example, only 40 per cent of the current attenders at day hospitals had a profile of needs that in our judgement warranted this form of intervention; 25 per cent would have been more appropriately placed in some form of out-patient care, such as follow-up care by a psychiatrist, community psychiatric nurse or, less often, a social worker or clinical psychologist.[19]

Conclusion

This chapter has reviewed the results of research which are of direct use to planners in that they indicate there is a range of unmet needs, many of which were directly identified by the individual client, that could have been alleviated by relatively small changes in existing practices or use of resources. However, it would be naive to argue that the orientation of planning in the future could be solely determined by the surveying of consumer needs. Clients do not speak with one voice; nor do they have the same problems. Indeed, they may well have competing problems, so that acting in some patients' interests may be detrimental to others or alienate some people in the local neighbourhood to which they may be returning. Furthermore, any conceivable organizational structure for delivering mental health care will impose its own set of constraints that must be accommodated in the planning process.

Less reassuring is the evidence that psychiatric services are still fostering dependency. Within present structures the promotion of patient autonomy is not guaranteed: for, though the 'enabling' role is increasingly being espoused in mental health care, one should not forget that psychiatry is entrusted with control functions, too, and sometimes these roles cannot be reconciled in practice. Finally, there is, as ever, the thorny issue of reconciling the interests of the user with those of the wide range of providers, whose professional socialization may well have encouraged a 'dependency' mentality and who, with the real threat to jobs in the psychiatric services, may have every reason to fear what the promotion of patient autonomy may mean for their future.

Note

I should like to thank Chris Brewin and Brigid MacCarthy of the MRC Social Psychiatry Unit for their helpful comments about earlier drafts of this paper.

Research of relatives' views has also been carried out by Brigid MacCarthy as part of the research outlined above but is not reported here.

References

1. Short Report (1985) *Second Report of the Social Services Committee,* HMSO, London.
2. Marshall, T.H. (1981) *The Right to Welfare,* Heinemann, London.
3. Foucault, M. (1973) *The Birth of the Clinic,* Tavistock, London.
4. Watts, F.N. & Bennett, D.H. (1983) *Theory and Practice of Rehabilitation,* Wiley, Chichester.
5. Wolfensberger, W. (1982) *Normalisation: The Principle of Normalisation in Human Services,* National Institute for Medical Research, Toronto.
6. Brandon, D. (1981) *Voices of Experience: Consumer Perspectives on Psychiatric Treatment,* MIND Publications.
7. King's Fund Centre (1977) *Psychiatric Hospitals Viewed by their Patients.*
8. Freeman, J. et al. (1965) 'Attitudes to Discharge Among Long Stay Mental Hospital Patients and their Relation to Social and Clinical Factors', *British Journal of Social and Clinical Psychology,* 4, pp. 270–4.

9. McCowan, P., Wilder, J. (1975) *Lifestyle of 100 Psychiatric Patients*, Psychiatric Rehabilitation Association Publications; (1983) *What Chance Have We Got*, MIND.

10. Pryce, I. et al. (1983) 'A Study of Long-Attending Psychiatric Day Patients and the Services Provided for them', *Psychological Medicine*, 13, pp. 875–84.

11. Bender, M. et al. (1981) 'Perceived Atmosphere in Day Units: A Consumer Oriented Research Study', *New Directions for Psychiatric Day Services*, MIND Publications.

12. Ross, G. (1981) *Lifestyle of Long-Term Psychiatric Patients in the London Borough of Hackney*, Psychiatric Rehabilitation Association.

13. Wykes, T. (1982) 'A Hostel-Ward for "New" Long-stay Patients', in Wing, J.K., Morris, B. (ed) *Handbook of Psychiatric Rehabilitation*, OUP, Oxford.

14. Wykes, T., Creer, C., Sturt, E. (1982) 'Needs and the Deployment of Services', Wing, ibid.

15. Sturt, E., Wykes, T., Creer C. (1982) 'Demographic, Social and Clinical Characteristics of the Sample', Wing, ibid.

16. MacCarthy, B., Benson, J., Brewin, C. (1988) 'Task Motivation and Problem Appraisal in Long Term Psychiatric Patients', *Psychological Medicine* (in press).

17. Frankham, D. 'Client Demand for Occupational Therapy Programmes' (in preparation).

18. Brewin, C. et al. (1988) 'Assessment of Need in the Long Term Mentally Ill', The Camberwell High Contact Study (in preparation).

19. Mangen, S. et al. (1988) *Service Implications of Needs in a Long-Term Day Care Clientele* (in preparation).

Address for information on the Camberwell studies still in preparation: Steen Mangen, MRC Social Psychiatry Unit, Institute of Psychiatry, De Crespigny Park, London SE5 8AF.

6

Towards a Rehabilitative Psychiatry

PAOLO HENRY

Editor's Introduction

This chapter is based primarily on the author's experience in Turin. It deserves our attention as an example of what can happen in a large conurbation. Turin has 1,200,000 inhabitants, many of whom immigrated from the Italian South during the boom years of the 1950s and the 1960s. It is one of Italy's most industrialized centres, with the Fiat complex as its symbol. It also has a history of a well-developed trade union movement and had an active anti-Fascist resistance movement during the Second World War. Today Turin has a very high unemployment rate and a crushed trade union movement. In the last local elections (June 1985) control of the city council moved from the Left to the Centre.

In the early 1970s Turin had about 4,500 in-patients, most of them in two nearby hospitals, Collegno and Grugliasco. Today there are no in-patients in Grugliasco, though 100 ex-patients live on the premises. Four hundred people are still patients in Collegno, about 1,000 ex-patients live in communities on the site and the rest are now living outside.[1] Part of the hospital is used as offices for the largest co-operative of ex-patients in Italy, with 170 members, which is a flourishing economic enterprise.[2] A day centre which offers an art workshop and cultural activities is available too on the site, together with a theatre workshop. The workshop is well known throughout the country because of an acclaimed play directed by the famous Russian director, Tarkovsky, which it produced with ex-patients.

The largest part of the old hospital site is used as a public park, with recreation areas for different games used by ordinary citizens. In the city there is a centralized facility for ex-patients, the Turin Project, which offers various vocational courses and recreation activities.

The latest development in the attempt to promote further the level of autonomy of those who live in the communities on the hospitals' sites is the one reflected upon by Paolo Henry below. Since January 1985 each community in Grugliasco has its own joint bank account, two elected representatives who can issue cheques, a centralized food and basic household materials shop, a centralized coffee place run by residents and an association called 'Spring 85' to which residents can affiliate, but do not have to do so. The bank, which provided the basic training for those authorized to issue cheques, has been surprised with the pace at which these people, each of whom has been in the psychiatric hospital for more than ten years, were able to learn the details of modern use of the banking system.

As could have been predicted, the main resistance to this move came from the ex-nurses of the psychiatric hospital who were responsible for the everyday running of the communities up to this point. They are losing power and part of their role through this change and unless they can redefine their tasks and achieve a sense of satisfaction from their redefined role, they will continue to sabotage the new regime.

Instead of the psychiatric hospital, there are five mental health centres in Turin itself with parallel 15-bedded units in five general hospitals. Several of the MHCs also have therapeutic communities attached, run day centres and a multitude of social, cultural and therapeutic activities. As can be expected, there are considerable variations in the philosophy and way of running the centres together with a number of unsatisfactorily resolved issues (such as housing). But nowhere is there a hankering for a *good psychiatric hospital*.

Shulamit Ramon

As the chief administrator of 'the residual' (as it is mercilessly but aptly defined) of what used to be three mental hospitals – now reorganized into nine communities in the social/health area of the Grugliasco ex-mental hospital – I am made aware daily and with increasing frequency how inadequate are both organic psychiatry and psychoanalysis in everyday practice.

Psychoanalytical and organic models of interpretation contradict each other only on the surface. In fact, they are based partly on shared assumptions of the qualitative difference between 'ill' and 'healthy' people. They both guarantee individual (imaginary) and positive (merely corporal) attention. This artificial model of man is in danger of separating and screening the reality of the actual individual in question. This is especially so if that individual is an ex-patient of a mental hospital who has to be 'rehabilitated'.

Like Physiotherapists?

Our work is like that of those involved in the physical rehabilitation of, say, patients who have suffered a heart attack, or old people who are bedridden after a bone fracture. Modern physiotherapy requires a tiring and painful rehabilitative routine. It aims at a return to normal movement. Often the return is hardly credible (at least at the beginning) and is therefore almost unwanted by the patient himself as well as his relatives.

The analogy between the rehabilitation of a long-stay psychiatric patient and physical rehabilitation has other parallels. Both treatments are characterized by an increase in pain and often a worsening of the symptoms in the initial stages of the rehabilitation process. However, the most interesting common factor is that even in the case of physical rehabilitation it is becoming increasingly obvious that scientific models of the clinical/pathological type are inadequate.

For example, in the case of a hemiplegic, knowledge of the mechanisms which caused the patient's imbalance is, in the end, of little importance. What is fundamentally valuable is knowing the mechanical and above all the neurophysiological functions of a healthy person's motor patterns. In fact, too much emphasis on the malfunctions of circulation can retard or diminish a patient's achievement of normal movement with harmful consequences for the patient's health as a whole.

As in psychiatry, in this case also, prognosis must take greater account of environmental factors (social conditions, family structure, work conditions, type of housing) than of 'endogenetic' factors.

Any successful attempt at the overall planning of an ex-patient's life bears little relation to the quantitative characteristics of conventional mental pathology. Therefore, it becomes even more evident how useless clinical diagnosis must be (based more or less on the traditional description of 'illness') in the case of patients who have been in mental hospitals for decades. A purely clinical approach is often paralysing in itself; the more so, if (as is happening increasingly) it is the 'maddest' people who ask (consciously or not) to 'go out'. Clinically speaking, they are the most serious cases and therefore the least suitable for discharge. On the other hand, elderly ex-patients no longer wish to leave. They have adjusted well mentally (so much so that they could be defined as 'cured') now that conditions in the former hospitals have improved and have been organized into more humane, 'autonomous-family' communities. If we do not succeed in motivating in them the desire for a more ordinary life, they could well remain within the confines of the ex-hospitals forever. This is because, contrary to the clinical approach, we believe that one of the various civil rights which they have acquired is the right not to be deported back, against their will, to other places which we, the new professionals, consider 'more suitable' for their treatment.

The Pinel–Itard debate at the End of the Eighteenth Century

As often happens the above contradiction, which some may believe they discovered after Law 180 came into effect in 1978, has ancient origins.

What seems to me to be particularly topical when comparing these models from the past is the paralysing impotence of Pinel's clinical approach when contrasted to Itard's optimistic approach.[3] Even though Itard was not certain he would completely achieve his stated objective, he began his rehabilitation work and achieved moderate success. In fact what interested the first 'professional re-educator' was not so much illness in the clinical sense as the social future of the person in question.

Even in its beginnings, clinical teaching had to take account of an educational model already in existence. At that time this model was beginning to change from being more or less ascientific to being more exact and enlightened. But within the space of a century the medicalization of psychic disorder was inappropriately monopolizing every type of deviation: from madness to dementia, from homosexuality to delinquency, from drug dependency to prostitution. This total monopoly was to be extended ever more inappropriately from treatment to prevention and then to rehabilitation. Law 180 lays down basic conditions for breaking with this monopoly.

When Pathology has an Iatrogenic Effect

Even if rehabilitation is difficult, the fact that handicap can be overcome increases society's duty to do so. But what remains of the 'pathogenic ailment' which originally led to a person's admission after 10, 20, 30 years inside a mental hospital? How is it possible to distinguish between the assumed 'illness' and the dramatic effects which medicalization and prolonged hospitalization will have had on a specific social case?

Take the example of an ex-patient who, say, refuses to manage her/his money or who will not turn out the lights at night. Does it make sense to ask whether this anomaly has been produced by the original intrapsychiatric process, or by the conditioning of institutional life or by more recent defence mechanisms?

It is scientifically impossible as well as entirely useless to know how much an ex-mental patient's social inadequacy is due to the original 'illness' or how much to long hospitalization. It stands to reason then (and is confirmed in practice) that any therapeutic process which does not plan a patient's life overall – as well as being healing and rehabilitative – is entirely useless.

In order to really 'treat' a patient properly, it must be necessary to support and aim for de-institutionalization, even if institutions have greatly improved in human terms.

In this way, a patient's use of time, his or her own home, work, belongings, management of his/her own property will change from being *signals* or *instruments* of a cure to being the *essence* of that cure. The essential value for human personality which they represent for most people will be acquired by 'mad' people also.

The Miracles of the Non-Specialists

The comparative powerlessness of clinical models is even more apparent when many psychotherapists (even the most eminent) confirm with guilty certainty that most long-stay patients are incurable. Given this, it is understandable that the representatives of the establishment's scientific community are amazed (even denying the evidence itself!) at the success achieved in this field by workers who sometimes have almost no formal clinical training.

Examples of these 'miracles' performed by non-specialists are becoming more and more numerous, and they include communities which are often managed by the unqualified staff of the old mental hospitals in a highly improvised manner, and who manage rather well despite a multitude of difficulties; and worker and/or service co-operatives, managed by workers on state-supported pay and sometimes even by ex-patients themselves.

Some 'progressive' psychiatrists who have witnessed the validity of these structures at first hand have used the phrase 'non-professional' for some of these miraculous, improvising workers. It is as if somehow the totally unexpected results have been achieved by accident; as if they did not indicate that a new type of professional had emerged and that there was an urgent need for the use of new scientific categorization.

What often happens is that teaching 'specialists' recycle their obsolete information in order to control and reduce the risk of subversion for the ruling established scientific community, while what should be taking place is the creation of a new basic theory using the systematic validation and comparison of these new successful working practices.

Which One of 'The Sane Person's' Psychologies?

When the 'New Co-operative' of Collegno and the 'Project Co-operative' of Turin – both of which are very experienced in training courses for long-stay psychiatric patients – had to choose the support method most suitable for their courses, it was no coincidence that the most useful indicators were not to be found among the varied and numerous instances of group therapy. Instead they were found in the experiments used by 'People Culture' during the French resistance to the German occupation when they focused on the issue of what type of society people wanted after the revolution; in the UNESCO programmes for disinherited South American peasants for self help in the eradication of poverty; in the pilot experiments in Turin among immigrants in the ghettos, and in the experiments for organizing trade unions there. It is interesting to note that in all of these learning processes, the concept of *consciousness* reacquires the meaning which was prevalent before psychoanalysis (which reduces it to a minor phenomenon of the unconscious) and achieves ideological predominance. It reacquires its original meaning – being the central element in regulating behaviour. Consciousness – that is, the new model for interpreting one's own environment – can only be measured by changes in behaviour.

A few years ago, I was lucky enough to take part in a professional training meeting for ex-mental patients. As members of a co-operative, they were organizing themselves to take on a large contract of cleaning a public building in Turin.

The 'gravity' of the pathology of some of them and, above all, my training as a group therapist made me particularly incapable of orientating myself. That strange meeting could have been seen as a professional training session for the use of new cleaning machinery; or as an important decision-making meeting for co-operative workers; or even as a collective psychotherapy session where the desires and fears of the participants (which were either expressed excitedly or by silences) were channelled into work plans by the psychotherapy leader.

But was the leader of that strange meeting really a psychotherapist or an able professional instructor? Or even the chairperson of a meeting of rather special co-operative workers? However, the 'anomaly' and the revolutionary contradictions of the situation did not exist in the actual experience of the participants. It was my previous mental constraints which made it difficult for me to understand its obvious simplicity. Perhaps at the beginning of the struggle against institutionalization it was not necessary to seek out new psychological models.

In the initial stages of liberating both workers and patients in the mental hospitals, models of sociopolitical consciousness were sufficient; or even models of 'commonsense psychology' which had been created by one's own family experience as a child or parent.

Now that the impetus of ideological struggle has ceased, we find ourselves in a much more difficult phase even though in many respects it is a much more advanced one. The family model now seems to have exhausted its potential for hospital culture, and demonstrates increasingly the limitations of its protective-maternal approach.

The communities which were the main instruments of anti-institutional struggle ten years ago are in danger of becoming the 'fetish' of new and more acceptable social control.

If progressive professionals continue to exhaust their educational capabilities in isolated and idealistic analyses, and if less-trained basic workers continue to use the psychology acquired from family experience, then even the new communities are in danger of becoming routine institutions, now that the initial impetus and enthusiasm experienced during the move from mental hospital wards to small communities has been lost. The large number of cases of successful rehabilitation is in danger of representing the limit of professional capabilities.

Proposals for the Future

It is for this reason that I am currently referring to existing schools of thought which might be useful for theoretical support in continuing a process initiated 20 years ago, and which have not been used up to now.

The first is *environmental psychology*, which originated in the US and arose out of joint urban planning work. The theoretical model in use derives particularly from a proposal put forward by Ivor Oddone[4] regarding the recovery of professional behaviours. The behavioural model for rehabilitators and rehabilitated should be the one formulated by Miller, Galanter and Pribani. With Hickson[5] they emphasize that the means by which the environment determines behaviour is one's perception of the environment.

The second is a model of personality structure used for biographical analysis of the *use of time*. This model is based on the Marxist hypothesis that human personality is determined by history. Of course, if this is to be incorporated into the real working practices of psychological work, as Seve[6] suggests, then it needs to be developed further in relation to both theory and methodology using the experimental evidence which is already available. For the time being it has been more useful to us as a model for interpreting our work than as an indicator for new professional solutions.

The instructions to the second self[7] are much more effective and have already been successfully tested several times. This is another method invented by Oddone during his attempt to reinterpret employees' experience at Fiat Mirafiori. The employee who accepted the need to restructure his/her experience instructs his hypothetical second self so that he can change places with him. What this entails in fact is an inherent awareness for obtaining a written plan of actual work behaviour. These plans are real ones and are as distant as possible from an idealized model of desired or desirable behaviour. This method provides a fundamental element of training which is really based on work experience. These three proposals have a new, common perspective: they focus on understanding everyday life of normal people.

I am increasingly convinced that it is only after we have analysed the normal, everyday qualities of human existence that we can then turn to the exceptional and the diverse. This procedure will guarantee that psychological knowledge is based on observation of the healthy individual. Our approach to pathology and clinical teaching will then take health as its point of departure and will subsequently place it as the point of arrival and return.

References

1. Giacopini, D. (1985) 'Lo smantellamento di un manicomio: l'area socio sanitaria di Grugliasco', *Psichiatria-Informazione* no. 2, Turin.
2. Di Mascio, A. (1986), 'L'esperienza de la Nuova Cooperativa: da degente all'autogestione collettiva del lavoro', *Psichiatria/Informazione*.
3. Lane, H. (1977) *The Wild Boy of Aveyron*, Allen & Unwin, London.
4. Oddone, I. (1979) *Psicologia dell'ambiente – Fabbrica e territorio*, Giappichelli, Turin.
5. Miller, G.A. et al. (1960) *Plans and the Structure of Behaviour*, Holt, New York.
6. Seve, L. (1978) *A Marxist Theory of Personality*, Macmillan, London.
7. Oddone, I., Briante, D.E. (1980) *Psicologia del Lavoro, esperienza operaia e coscienza di classe*, Einaudi, Milan.

7

Ethnicity and Gender as Uncomfortable Issues

NAOMI SELIG

> It all started five years ago with terrible headaches from too much thinking, thinking, thinking. I knew he was seeing other women ... He came home drunk all the time. The doctors think I have depression. They gave me ECT but it made me sick. I have so much time in the house for thinking, thinking, it gets worse. When I get like this I just take my pills and want to sleep all the time. I can't cope with the housework and the children. If people talk to me I cry. I feel so lonely but I can't communicate. My husband thinks I am crazy because I have psychiatric treatment. I don't tell anyone else because they would think I am mad. They think madness is catching.[Asian woman]

This woman speaks for many who like her are receiving psychiatric treatment which does little to alleviate their distress. If anything, her sense of despair, of helplessness and personal inadequacy has increased over the years, even with psychiatric treatment. Contributing to her malaise is her relatively powerless position, both in relation to her husband, and as a member of an ethnic minority which is in itself oppressed. Unable to cope with an untenable situation, she is presumed to be ill – the fault is attributed to her. By giving authority to the notion that she is mad, psychiatric treatment perpetuates her subordination and isolation, both within her home and outside. She does not receive support and understanding from her own community, nor from the dominant culture. Her problems are compounded by her subordinate status, not only as a woman but also as a member of an ethnic minority – yet this is disregarded by everyone, even herself.

A sense of helplessness, hopelessness and lack of control over one's life features large in depression. However, these feelings may not be symptoms of an individual's psychopathology. Rather, they may be reality-based amongst people who have genuinely little power to influence their circumstances. Brown and Harris's[1] community study showed that a majority of working-class women with young children at home, who lacked intimacy in their relationships and had no outside employment, were particularly vulnerable to depression. Likewise, institutional racism and sexism imposes restrictions on its victims, for example, via racist employment practices; immigration laws which keep families apart; racist attacks – such events would certainly be provoking agents in depression.

The power structure of psychiatry itself is a prime example of how racism and sexism can be institutionalized. Most prestigious, powerful and 'clean' jobs, such as consultant psychiatrists, are occupied by white men. They have had a privileged education and, in the case of doctors, are often the offspring of doctors themselves. Descending the hierarchy in terms of power and pay, the 'mucky' jobs, such as nursing and cleaning, are occupied by working-class women who are often black, Asian, or Irish. Moreover, white men move up the hierarchy more quickly than women or men from ethnic minorities – not only because they are more likely to get the powerful jobs, but also because women and people from minority groups are less likely to apply for them.

Recently I was in a department in which a top grade psychology post was advertised. While there are actually more females in the profession, not a single woman applied. For one reason or another they felt they were not able, although their achievements to date would indicate the opposite. So even among relatively enlightened, educated women, this deep sense of inferiority, so prevalent among female patients, is often too great to shift.

Baker Miller[2] has argued that unequal power relationships are legitimated and incorporated into society's guiding concepts – its morality, philosophy, and science. Because it is institutionalized, inequality becomes obscured and is regarded as natural and normal. Our institutions reinforce the belief that the way things are is right and proper, not only for those with power, but also for those in subordinate roles. It then becomes possible to explain what happens in terms of such false premises as racial or sexual inferiority. While it is difficult for those in positions of power to believe their underlings could actually perform the preferred activities, worse still is the fact that those who are subordinated often share this belief.

Given the distribution of power in psychiatry it is not surprising that treatment offered reflects this and perpetuates the dominant ideology. But, as Althusser[3] says, 'ideology has very little to do with consciousness ... it is profoundly unconscious'. This is exemplified in a study conducted by Broverman and her associates in the US.[4] Seventy-nine male and female clinicians were divided into three groups, and each group was asked to fill out sex-role questionnaires describing either healthy, desirable characteristics of adult men, or adult persons, or adult females. Both male and female clinicians considered that the ideal characteristics of an adult male did not differ significantly from those of an adult person. However healthy women differed from a healthy person or healthy man by being

> more submissive, less independent, less adventurous, more easily influenced, less aggressive, less competitive, more excitable in minor crises, having their feelings more easily hurt, more emotional, less objective, and more conceited.

Paradoxically then, women cannot be both healthy adults and healthy women. If they fit the stereotype for the healthy adult they are deemed unfeminine. But if they fit the stereotype for the healthy female they are socially inadequate and would be entirely incapable of coping with the demands of the world we live in. This non-coping being is an implicit model clinicians use in assessing female patients. If women coming into hospital are viewed in such terms, should they then be helped to regain the status of a healthy woman, or would this not condemn them to further subordination?

Similar stereotypes are operative in relation to ethnic minority groups. For example, 'happy-go-lucky, lazy, simple and childish' may be considered normal characteristics for a black or Irish person. But if they are angry they are deemed maladjusted and deviant, even though this often seems appropriate in the context. If they are not 'mad' they are 'bad' – the prison population demonstrates this.

Psychiatric labelling locates the disorder within the individual's pathology rather than within the system which oppresses such individuals. Despite the fact that in Britain one in every five women takes tranquillizers, that twice as many women than men receive treatment for 'affective' disorders, and that of these, five times as many are likely to be working class than middle class; none of these statistics have really been subjected to political scrutiny which could lead to social change.

But labels too have their hierarchy. For instance, black people are generally not regarded by clinicians as even suffering from depression, although they may be called schizophrenic.[5] Could it be that the age-old image that 'primitives' are not sophisticated enough to feel depressed persists? Perhaps inertia and hopelessness, recognized as characteristic of depression, is in black people regarded as laziness, obstinacy, or even stupidity?

I have heard a consultant psychiatrist justify a virtually non-existent service provision for Asians by saying that they did not suffer from psychological problems. This was in a catchment area where Asians form one of the largest ethnic minority groups. No enquiry has been made as to the validity of such a statement in this area, presumably because it is not considered worthwhile. Evidence would suggest however that people from the Asian community avoid psychiatric services because they recognize that, for the most part, what they would be offered would be worse than nothing, and the stigma of a psychiatric label would be too much to bear.[6]

So-called 'liberal' doctors are now beginning to pay lip-service to the dangers of cultural hegemony in psychiatric practice, but use this recently acknowledged information in a way which unwittingly oppresses people further. Just as Broverman and her colleagues showed that what is considered 'normal' by clinicians for healthy women is synonymous with helpless, non-coping beings, there are analogies with respect to race and culture. Intolerable practices are regarded as 'normal' for a particular culture and therefore exonerated. The following illustrations exemplify this.

Recently I was asked to assess an extremely distressed Jewish woman on a locked ward who had attempted suicide during her pregnancy. The nurse said that through her pregnancy the woman had shared a bed with her father, and that when her father visited they engaged in intimate embraces of an apparently sexual nature. When the nurse tentatively suggested to the consultant psychiatrist that perhaps this was an incestuous relationship, the psychiatrist replied that on the contrary, such affection was normal among Jews. The question of incest as a factor in her distress would therefore not be addressed.

Similarly there are instances where male psychiatrists encourage Muslim women to return to their violent husbands, because this is alleged to be normal practice. This combination of racism and sexism, when cloaked in 'liberalism', can be even harder to identify and is therefore even more pernicious. Fernando[7] has shown how the three main components of depression/low self-esteem, a sense of loss and a sense of helplessness can be induced by racism.

If people from a subordinated group internalize the values of the dominant social groups, they will believe that they are inferior and inadequate. Furthermore, this inferior status is considered permanent if it is attributed to immutable characteristics, such as race or sex. The following vignette may illustrate how this process happens.

In a conversation with a powerful colleague who regards herself as 'liberal', I explained that although not at all religious, I felt and identified myself as Jewish. She told me that I must surely be mistaken, because Jews are mean and she liked me. She then rationalized this by suggesting that perhaps I was an exceptional Jew. The implication of all this was that I was either identifying with a mean, unscrupulous group of people or I was not really a proper Jew. But I was not anything else either. If I were to believe her I would experience conflict, confusion, and alienation.

This is a very crude example – consider the pernicious effect of years of experiencing such devaluation of your cultural background, and/or your gender, subtly reinforced by institutional practices. As Fernando says,

> It is not culture as some theoretical concept that is devalued in a racist society; it is the person himself who is devalued including his skin colour, his mannerisms, and often his way of life. If these sorts of values are incorporated by (for example) a black person, he could be said to 'hate' his black identity and have low self esteem.[8]

Similarly, Sartre[9] wrote about the anti-Semitic Jew who 'is poisoned by the stereotype that others have of him'.

The low self-esteem manifest in the majority of women is instilled by similar processes.

Fernando argues that a sense of loss, to which I would add a sense of personal inadequacy, is likely to occur in a society which does not acknowledge that institutional racism (or sexism) contributes to the thwarting of everyday achievements and rewards. He considers this in the context of anti-Semitism and depression among Jews in East London. In a culture which promotes the expectation of achievement in proportion to merit, a person who expects to get something and then does not (be it a job, exam or visa) is likely to feel angry (through frustration) and 'less' of the object which in his fantasy he actually had. He argues that failure to achieve in line with norms is a kind of loss. It is well nigh impossible for many people in subordinate roles to achieve in line with activities which are valued by and protected by those of the dominant cultural groups. When people blame themselves for their lack of achievement or loss, rather than recognizing its cause as external they are more vulnerable to depression.

For treatment to be effective in helping people from oppressed groups, it is necessary to acknowledge in treatment the relationship between institutional practices such as racism and sexism, and the psychology of the individual.

Fernando has considered the implications of low self-esteem in treatment. He maintains it is essential to acknowledge the blows to self-esteem arising from racism. When people from oppressed groups have sufficient sources of self-pride to draw on, they tend not to introject the negative values from the dominant culture. As Kapo[10] says, 'The identity of anyone *aware* of being a victim is always clear cut.'

Fernando suggests that perhaps this is why Jews have often managed to maintain self-esteem through generations of anti-Semitism, and why strong ethnic links often arise among ethnic minorities in racist societies. Similarly, feminist women are less likely to accept and internalize the negative male attributes considered appropriate for their sex.

Strategies to safeguard self-esteem and alternative sources of pride must be sought, for example, by identifying (if black) with black movements, seeking ethnic therapists, or finding models that do not represent the dominant groups. Moreover, Fernando argues that if the replenishment of self-esteem cannot be sustained through normal channels, so-called deviant behaviour may be the only way of bolstering self-esteem. For example, while neighbourhood vigilante groups or social self-assertion may be desirable, rioting may be more appropriate if other ways of self-assertion are blocked.

The therapist should be aware of the subtle effects of racism when dealing with a client's sense of loss. Conventional approaches in which patients are encouraged to 'come to terms' and 'work through' their loss, and lower expectations, is not helpful. Facilitating anger and action against future losses is probably more therapeutic. Similarly, patients who feel they have no control over their lives should not be told to accept their condition – as Valium-filled women are expected to do – but should be encouraged to develop strategies for self-assertion and control over events. It is vital that clinicians identify racism and sexism as the restrictive yoke which so often prevents clients from controlling their environment, thereby leading to ways of encouraging resistance and self-assertion.

It is essential that therapists recognize the ethnocentric and sexist values implicit in conventional approaches. For instance, while individual therapy can be helpful, an emphasis on individual growth and self-actualization which does not take into consideration the position of the individual within their own social group, and their obligations and loyalties, may be culturally an anathema. A cognitive therapist, for example, should be aware of racist value judgements when assessing what is viable or rational. Even when a client feels in conflict about their roles and obligations this does not mean that they wish to relinquish their own cultural values, nor applaud English individualism.

Central to the place of gender and ethnicity in everyday psychiatric practice is the issue of power. It is questionable whether real or enduring change can be achieved without a transformation of the power structure of psychiatry, and more broadly, society at large. There is a persuasive argument, advocated by those of the anti-psychiatry movement, for ignoring psychiatry altogether, because by its very nature it merely perpetuates and endorses the status quo. I am of the opinion that if possible, it is better not to throw out the baby with the bath water – in other words, it may be possible to retain some of the better features of the psychiatric system. At any rate, it exists and affects thousands of people, who will continue to be affected unless the system itself is tackled.

In Britain the current state of the transcultural psychiatry movement is at a crossroads. There are broadly two camps: first those who consider the central issue to be racism, over and above cultural and ethnic differences, and second, those who regard culture and ethnicity as crucial, but who in my opinion lack a political perspective – power is not an issue they contend with. The movement started some 15 years ago, when white liberal consultant psychiatrists working in areas with diverse ethnic populations began to acknowledge that there were different manifestations of 'psychiatric illness' among people of different ethnic groups. Prior to this, transcultural psychiatry reflected the colonial stance, manifest for example in the mass of epidemiological studies which looked at the incidence of schizophrenia and other psychiatric syndromes across the world. Differences and similarities were found, but, willy-nilly, all findings were used to endorse a classification system which basically 'proved' that English public school boys really were better, saner, and more intelligent than the weaker sex, and the 'primitives' from the nether regions.

Tentatively, more enlightened doctors, influenced by the humanistic and anti-psychiatry movement, began to question the universality of their diagnoses. However for them there was never any question of the actual validity of the psychiatric model, merely that people could be misdiagnosed if their cultural background was not accounted for. Attempts were made, in both the North and South of England, to recruit people with the same ethnic background as their clients, who would be better able to communicate and form accurate diagnoses and treatment plans. But the power relationship between practitioners, and practitioners and clients, remained unchallenged, and the psychiatric model unquestioned. An important consequence of this change of practice among people with high status and respect, is that it legitimized and sanctioned the notion that one must respect cultural and ethnic differences. Television caught on to the bandwagon, books were published, and there was now a new angle on the magic of madness. The black person next door who seems to be freaking out may not be mad, but may be displaying some weird religious practice that they do where they come from.

To show how really concerned everyone is, there is now the token lecture in the training of doctors, nurses, social workers and, more recently still, psychologists, on the importance of culture and ethnicity in psychiatric practice. The message is that if you read the recipe book of different cultural groups, you will make the correct diagnosis. Bear in mind, for instance, that Jews and Muslims have dietary customs; their refusal to eat pork may not be a sympton of psychopathology. Recognize that people from different social backgrounds have different family structures, and their psychopathology reflects the fact that, indeed, these systems do cause them to be ill. The racist myths persist under the liberal veneer – so Jewish men who come into contact with psychiatry have problems because of 'over-intrusive' Jewish mothers, and Afro-Caribbean men are perceived as having problems because of 'negligent' black mothers. In this current 'liberal' atmosphere, the crux of the matter, racism, and in the case of women, sexism – is ignored or at best is paid lip-service.

In opposition to this liberal stance are those who also work within psychiatry and in community based groups, largely from the lower echelons of the power structure, and more often than not from black and ethnic minority groups. They regard racism as the overriding cause of mental problems for clients from black and ethnic minority groups. While I agree this is crucial, I do not think racism, or sexism, is necessarily the root of all ills. It is vital however that therapists are sensitive to its pernicious effects and ensure this is brought into treatment. Hopefully this is not at the expense of hearing other problems a client may have which may not be directly attributable to racist, sexist or sexual abuse. Having recognized the importance of these issues, the main problem for politically and self-aware practitioners is not how one approaches these issues in individual therapy, but how one tackles these issues at large.

Across the country different groups are dealing with this question in ways that seem most appropriate or viable for them. In the North London borough where I work, which comprises people of diverse cultural and ethnic origins, we have recently started an ongoing group which focusses on transcultural and racist issues within the mental health services. About 30 of us, from a range of disciplines and positions in the hierarchy, meet on a regular basis outside work to explore issues of power and racism within our practice. Aside from the more long-term objectives of changing practice and structure, initiating research and pressing for service developments and improvements, we consider self-awareness and the issue of power and racism between workers as primary. We aim to avoid simplistic approaches to this whole area and also the feelings of hopelessness and inertia that the awareness of racism can engender, particularly among white people. A central problem, yet to be tackled, is how we can be more effective in the long term. There is obvious resistance in the establishment to anything more than token gestures, which suggests practice may be less than perfect.

Ultimately, these groups need to become a political force to be reckoned with, so that health authorities, like some education authorities, adopt anti-racist policies for both employment and practice. This is hard to envisage in the present, increasingly reactionary, political climate.

References

1. Brown G., Harris T. (1978) *The Social Origins of Depression*, Tavistock Press, London.
2. Baker Miller, J. (1976) *Toward a New Psychology of Women*, Pelican Books, London.
3. Althusser, L. (1969) *For Marx*, Allen Lane Press, London.
4. Broverman I., Broverman D., Clarkson F., Rosenkrauts P., Vogel, S. (1970) 'Sex-Role Stereotypes and Clinical Judgements of Mental Health', *Journal of Consulting and Clinical Psychology*, 34, pp. 1–7.
5. Littlewood R., Lipsedge M. (1982) *Aliens and Alienists*, Penguin, Harmondsworth.
6. Selig N. (1981) 'Asians and Psychiatry', unpublished thesis, University of Leeds; Selig, N. (1983) 'White Magic', *Changes* (psychology and psychotherapy journal).
7. Fernando, S. (1984) 'Racism as a Cause of Depression', *International Journal of Social Psychiatry*, 30, 1 and 2.
8. ibid.
9. Sartre, J.P. (1948) *Antisemite and Jew*, Schocken Books, New York.
10. Kapo, R. (1981) *A Savage Culture*, Quartet Books, London.

8

Gender in the Italian Services

MARIA GRAZIA COGLIATI, SILVANA PETRI,
MARIA TERESA PINI

This chapter is focused on the impact of gender within the work of the health and mental health services.

Unlike in Britain, ethnicity is not a central issue in present-day Italy. However, internal migration of people from the south to the north, from one social class to another and from a traditional to a modern society is an issue which will be reflected in this chapter in its relationship to gender.

Concerning Italy's largest ethnic minority – the Slovene people – *Psichiatria Democratica* (PD) always took the position of treating its members as equal to other Italians. Furthermore, when they were threatened by Italian Fascists in the 1970s, PD members in Trieste – a city with a significant component of Slovenes – participated in a demonstration where the main slogan was 'We are all Slovenes!'

PD has given specific thought to the relationships between gender and health and between women and psychiatric practice. The examples of current practice described below come from a family planning unit near Naples and from a mental health centre in Trieste.

The experience of restructuring the psychiatric hospitals in the 1960s and 1970s (described in Chapters 16, 18 and 20) demonstrated that this social institution was more violent and repressive towards women than men. In the process of depersonalization exercised on all patients, strict separation by gender took place. This measure led to the suspension of all social roles. In addition, any manifestation of sexual desire on the part of female patients was stigmatized as obscene, and castigated as behaviour to be repressed. Relatively harsh measures were used for repression, such as confinement to bed, while at the same time cases of masculine masturbation were widely tolerated. Similarly, the existence of homosexual relations in male wards was tolerated without constraint while the same behaviour in female wards attracted the most rigorous taboo.

This is why one of the first objectives of the PD movement was the reconstruction of sexual identity. Attention was paid to caring for the body and physical appearance. Opportunities were provided both inside and outside the institution where both sexes could meet.

However, the specific nature of the female condition presented itself even more clearly when the reasons for admission were examined and when work outside the institution began to increase. Being in contact with the type of psychiatric disorders common to women before their admission has enriched our understanding of and ability to respond to the issues at stake.

On the one hand, it was observed[1] that deviant behaviour leading to psychiatric admission was usually proposed for women on the basis of their gender behaviour, while for men this happened in only a minority of cases. On the other hand it was notable, and still is, how widespread experiences of guilt, self-punishment and self-denigration are presented in the form of 'madness' in women.

In principle, psychiatric textbooks agree that women's psychiatric disorders are related to a refusal or incapacity to respond to their own social role in both its sexual and domestic aspects. Of course, the way in which these doctors have interpreted this 'non-respect', i.e. the way in which they identify the individual's value and how they expect it to affect their prognostic evaluation, does not correspond to the interpretation made by the women's movement or that of the PD (for the analysis of traditional psychiatry regarding women, see Chesler).[2]

Not respecting the sexual role is viewed traditionally as a self-destructive reaction which is completely subjective. Even if it manifests itself by considerably diverse symptoms, it allows a certain number of disorders, all connected with feelings of guilt and inadequacy, to be grouped together. Female disorders are usually related to the following clinical definitions: depression, anxiety, frigidity, psychoneurosis, suicide attempts.

The feminist interpretation has highlighted the subjective reaction to an objective condition of impotence and lack of power. The forms of expression mentioned above are recognized as developments, however grotesque at times, of the very characteristics of the female sexual role, such as passivity, loss of identity and self-depreciation.

In circumstances where this non-response is countered by a denial of these 'feminine' characteristics as well as an active denial of the sexual role, more 'masculine' disorders can be observed, namely aggression and activity against the accepted moral code resulting in schizophrenia, lesbianism, promiscuity.

But whatever the experience which accompanies 'madness', PD

practitioners have observed a common underlying thread in its patients' histories; a common denominator which embraces women of all classes, all generations and often different cultural contexts.[3] They are always reduced to being only bodies, or individuals living as a function of other members of the family, defined via others: wives in respect of husbands, daughters in respect of parents, mothers in respect of children.

Therefore, in a culture like ours, being sentenced to self-limitation and to alienation is inherent in the female condition. Every time women are examined in medicine or psychiatry, they are judged according to roles and behaviour linked to their bodies or their families.

Why have women been reduced to these limited levels of action and expression – the body and the family? Why are all attempts to go beyond these limitations either explicitly repressed or accompanied by such guilt feelings as to usually lead to abandoning the crossing of the boundaries? One reason could be the masculine view of female biology in which a woman's body is all 'nature'. Its maturation stages, its gradual changes seem regulated by fixed periods, almost intrinsically imposed by its biology: menstruation, fertility cycles and menopause. Ideologically, the already simplified equation women's body = nature becomes extended, so that everything which women are today is so *because of nature*. That is to say, weak by nature, beautiful by nature, tender by nature, maternal by nature and so on. So anybody who is not weak, beautiful, tender or maternal *is unnatural* therefore morally culpable.

This framework explains why such models of femininity are widely internalized into the female psyche. It also explains the high price paid in terms of guilt feelings or 'malice' on the part of those who rebel.

In reality this rigid fixing of woman's image, justifying its feminine qualities through reference to natural biology, has one very distinct consequence: that of reducing women to the status of *bodies to be owned* both in the physical (a body to penetrate) and socioeconomic sense (being a subordinate and acquiescent individual).

All female attributes are subordinated to this image, leading to the following:

- A constant double message is given on female identity: the feminine gift of seduction is developed, at the expense of other human talents, and then it must be repressed or controlled to accommodate the demands of men or motherhood.
- Having to exist as a body *for others only* creates an internal rift in the female body: in erotic relationships women must create a distance between themselves and their bodies. They are then able to

experience it as an object for others. They must become objects in their own eyes to achieve this. They have to alienate themselves from their own bodies.

It will now be clear why in our culture attributes such as passivity, willingness to have one's body owned, giving, and negation of self in others are considered natural for women.

These attributes are considered ideal as regards women's mental health. They prescribe a precise, restrictive set of values in the permitted spheres of action such as sexuality within the family, motherhood and domestic activity on behalf of the family. Where a woman's control of this internalized set of values fails, she may impose upon herself a restriction on space (confinement to the house) or even have her sexuality forcibly controlled by being psychiatrized.

The following examples from the family advice centre demonstrate the internalization of the socially prescribed female identity and the price women pay for it. The description also outlines what can be done for women in such a service.

A.F., 32 years old, three children, two abortions, husband unemployed:

I don't want to use contraceptives. I am afraid they will harm me! ... But you run the risk of becoming pregnant again!
There's no danger of that. I know what to do.
The withdrawal method?
No, no! I know that's not safe. Well, anyway, I can tell you, we are amongst women. So that my husband is not frustrated, I masturbate him or else I let him have pleasure by putting it between my breasts.

There is embarrassment. It's difficult to give even a mundane reply. It is only during a successive meeting that we are able to ask:

So you never experience pleasure?
I don't know what that is. I don't mind. The most important thing is that my husband is calm and I don't get pregnant again.

Everything is contained in this account – loneliness, resignation, violence. Her own sexuality and body are overcome and absorbed by having to be first and foremost a wife and mother who must satisfy other people's needs exclusively.

S.P., 27 years old, two children, and uses the pill. We have known her since she came during her first pregnancy. She has a very pleasant appearance and dresses in the latest fashion; she is modern. She comes one day asking to speak urgently:

> Last night I felt a strange thing while I was with my husband, which
> I have never felt in my five years of marriage. I was frightened. It
> was almost painful.

After a long conversation, it was discovered that this strange thing was
none other than an orgasm. She did not recognize it. She had never even
heard of it and she is afraid of feeling this sensation again. She is
lonely. She has no friends because 'the children and the house keep me
busy all day.'

C.P., 39 years old, plain appearance, almost scruffy, does not show any
particular care for her clothes or for her body. She had a coil fitted by us
two years ago. She has had three children, one abortion, and has come
to have the IUD removed and replaced with another. She is advised for
gynaecological reasons to wait two months before having the new one
fitted. She is told that in the meantime her husband can use sheaths

> But my husband is already using them. You see, I don't know how to
> put this, but you will understand me, I've known another man for some
> time who I make love to from time to time. With him I use the coil,
> with my husband the sheath, that way I avoid him catching
> infections from the other man. My husband has never known that I've
> had a coil fitted.

Woman's impure, corrupt body, home of secretions and of both physical
and moral contamination has always throughout history, theology,
language and culture been contrasted with the body of woman, giver of
life, sacred, pure, asexual mother.

There then was a prime consideration regarding our work: we
recognized that the women in that locality, because of their level of
education or feminine oppression, had no other way of expressing
themselves or their needs except by requesting 'neutral' medical
services; the opportunity for providing medical services therefore
became for our work the means (sometimes the most important) by which
situations of unexpressed disadvantage, fear and guilt emerged which
were determined without a doubt by the social role which the women
experienced in their socioeconomic environment.

On the one hand, this meant we had to assume an analytical view of
the obstetric-gynaecological request in order to uncover latent needs
which were more profound and also to change the request for services,
once met, into a desire for shared personal experiences or life conditions.

Since our everyday practice presented this opportunity during normal consultations we were able to listen to women expressing their need for reassurance or for escape from feelings of guilt or the sanctioning of their hidden desires. This we did so that these feelings were recognized as being worthy of existence as well as those needs of a more strictly technical nature which were already permissible.

On the other hand, we tried to facilitate spontaneous group socialization for sharing personal experiences by timetabling our work so that on particular days women with similar problems or needs were brought together. On a day in which consultation work took place all pregnant women, or all women with contraceptive problems, for instance, would find themselves together. The time spent waiting became quite easily an opportunity, while an all-female non-medical staff also was present, for talking about personal experiences, for receiving advice and opinions from others, in a certain sense for testing the solidarity of a group in similar circumstances, using as a point of departure the reason why each individual was there.

Carrino[4] maintains that identity is a social product created as 'an instrument inside the individual, which is internalized and made part of him/herself. It ensures that each one of us conforms to the dominant model of social organization.' This conceptual framework enabled us to trace private experiences back to social mechanisms. Instead of these being only individual or subjective phenomena, they become linked to class, to the historical context of a society's development.

This analysis has several consequences pertaining to female identity, in particular:

- Behaviour and experience linked to sexuality and the body in general (for example, the various signals of well-being or discontent now no longer acknowledged, understood or respected);
- Those linked to the reproductive function with its various problems of contraception, pregnancy and confinement;
- Those relating to problems of motherhood and the parenting role of the partner;
- Those of personality development and social identity during the formative years, often with dramatic problems of generation conflict.

As we have seen in relation to the work of the family planning team, these contextualized experiences linked to the body and the family become the material for analysis and treatment. They must in fact be put into their context. Connotations of 'naturalness' and therefore of the 'indisputable truth' have to be eliminated. Guilt feelings linked to the gap between the ideal model of femininity and the practical possibility of anyone adhering to and actually living according to this model must be challenged.

Established medicine and psychiatry carry therefore with them a cultural vision and an organization of responses which are doubly violent towards women: this is because of its underlying values (moralistic, respectable, afraid of sexuality, riddled with taboos and prejudice) and because of relationship structures typical of the health system.

A relevant argument, very dear to the feminist debate, is that teams who work in the health services with women should be made up exclusively of women. Giannelli[5] has demonstrated in her research that young women indeed prefer female doctors.

In our opinion – that is, PD – all-women teams are not a necessity. Ensuring a feminist perspective and feminist practice during consultations is, however, a must. Furthermore, while an all-women team in a family planning service is likely to cater adequately for its users' psychosocial needs, the desirability of an all-women team in a psychiatric service is doubtful. This is so because the service would stop being for all people and become selective, as would the responses. If the issue of a woman's identity in the world as it exists is to be resolved then her relationships to men need to be examined too. For this purpose the men working in a psychiatric service which accepts and respects the feminist perspective can provide for the women users a corrective experience by offering mutually respectful relationships. In addition, because of the segregation suffered by all users, we are against its reintroduction even if it is for more positive purposes.

This struggle against the technicalization and medicalization of health, together with criticism of the social attributes to women's role and personality stated above, contribute to the real prevention of female psychic disorder.

By responding to these problems within the context of mother-infant consultation, health education programmes in school, mental health intervention during the formative years (in other words by intervening before discontent is translated into psychiatric problems), the other great ideal of the feminist movement can be advanced in the only way possible for health services: that is, via collective consciousness, or better still, consciousness of a collective condition as a means of liberation.

At this level the woman who requests a contraceptive, or the adolescent girl who attends a course of sexual education, is primarily a female; she is an active and dignified individual who is potentially capable of using the collective nature of her condition to strengthen her positive identity. By contrast the point of departure in psychiatric practice is an experience of defeat, failure or incapability.

The task is long and complex. Its starting point must be the positive reconstruction of female identity. The work carried out with Anna, described below, demonstrates the principles and issues raised above.

Anna, a 40-year-old woman, was brought to Barcola Mental Health Centre (one of the seven centres in Trieste operating 24 hours a day referred to in Chapter 4) by a teacher from the summer school which she was attending with her 14-year-old-son. She was at the peak of a psychotic crisis: hallucinating, worried, insomniac. She would not eat because the food was 'poisoned'. She tried to escape because she felt seriously threatened. She attacked everybody because she feared being attacked. She arrived directly at the centre, not having been through the psychiatric emergency service.

She was born into a family of humble origins; through her marriage to a 'sea captain', she attempted and succeeded in a rapid social ascent. She left her job as a shop assistant, her friends, her council house and no longer spoke in the local dialect. She became the wife of a professional man and lived like one.

After several years the relationship broke down. Her husband left her for another woman. Anna, alone, without work, with a grown-up son and in bad economic circumstances, found herself with an identity crisis. The legal separation which terminated her role as 'wife of ...', also deprived her of her function and social class. It is difficult to fill such a deep void at the age of 40. And the crisis took place.

While in the mountains with her son, in a summer camp run by the seamen's organization, she comes up against opportunities, lifestyles, individuals which are no longer hers but which she very much wants. So she tries in a clumsy way to seduce one of the men present because she is not capable of controlling her anxious behaviour. The summer camp is shocked and frightened. Anna feels attacked. She is frightened and attacks back. She is led away and taken to the Barcola Mental Health Centre.

Thus the Barcola Mental Health Centre was confronted with her suffering – in this case, female suffering. What can be offered to her, particularly in a public structure such as a mental health centre which has replaced the mental hospital? Let's try to analyse whether it is possible to deal with female suffering in a public structure, staffed by both men and women, by offering a response which has been defined by women themselves.

Rather than dwelling on her fragile state or on the crisis of a precariously constructed identity we tried instead to discover her capabilities and the richness in her history to date. This demonstrated a desire for change and affirmed her individuality and capacity for autonomous expression.

The centre then did not propose either Anna's isolation, or the containment or elimination of her symptoms by abstracting her outside the continuity of her life's context, as would have happened in the traditional psychiatric approaches. Instead Anna was welcomed and protected, her crisis being interpreted as a phase in her life, closely linked to her past and conditioned by it. It was positively positioned and referred to in her current life-history and context as a source of new plans.

In her crisis, Anna was taken back home. She was helped to maintain her relationship with her son whom her husband wanted to take away; defended from the prejudice of her in-laws; helped to defend her property; helped to take care of her appearance; and looked after with kindness but also firmness when she attempted to offer her body (which was, after all, her only certainty at the time).

So using the resources available in the service – board and lodging, consultations, accompaniment, personal care, gymnastics, workshops, work rehabilitation, financial benefits and medication – Anna's search was directed. She accepted that she must rely on her own resources without anxiously seeking a solution to her problem in others. She began to look around, initiating new relationships. She gained confidence and faith in herself. She asked for help in finding work suited to her capabilities so that she no longer needed to depend completely on her husband.

As soon as her crisis was over, Anna began helping the elderly as suggested by the centre. She was also able to use one of the resources which the service offers – a financial benefit, designated for the recognition of work activities such as assisting others or self-help. Her newly-acquired identity, which is more stable and reassuring, is translated into newly-acquired economic power, various points of reference and various social relationships.

This is a positive contribution which at the time proved beneficial, even if it certainly did not provide a final solution. From a distance the Mental Health Centre continues to support her, makes life easier for her, protects her and encourages her to gradually acquire higher levels of independence.

In this case, introducing psychiatry was certainly not a risk to Anna's existence as a woman. It would have been more risky not to intervene and avoid the so-called psychiatrization. The intervention was a necessary step and the service correctly assumed responsibility. The ultimate aim was to support recovery, the acquisition and maintenance of greater, real autonomy by Anna, perhaps for the first time in her life.

References

1. Harrison, L. (1976) *Donne, povere, matte*, Edizioni delle Donne, Rome.
2. Chesler, P. (1972) *Women and Madness*, Doubleday, New York.
3. Basaglia, F. Ongaro (1977) 'Un Commento', in the Italian translation of Chesler's book (ibid.), Einaudi, Milan.
4. Carrino, L. (1968) *Identità sessuale e istituzione psichiatrica*, privately circulated.
5. Giannelli, M.T. (1981) *Il Sud della Donne*, Unicopli, Milan.

9

Marginalization of Users and Providers in Britain

ALEC JENNER

Marx and Engels wrote in The *Holy Family*:

> The propertied class and the class of the proletariat present the same human self-estrangement. But the former class feels at ease and strengthened in this self-estrangement, it recognizes estrangement as its own power and has in it the semblance of a human existence.[1]

The psychiatrically marginalized cannot use their 'alienation' (the 'false human relationship in which man stands to himself').[2] Instead it becomes a basis for compassion and coercion from the alienists.

I criticize British psychiatry as a part of it, and as one familiar with my own club. I do not castigate it to exonerate other professions, each of which has similar problems. The inevitable and personally necessary struggle of an individual to find his identity involves immersion in subgroups, as well as politeness and collusion.

All systems within which one can act well for the particular group and get commendation and love – the family, for example – can also damage. So much of life shows an inevitable need to settle for something between the extremes of individualism and corporatism. What is reasonable? The answer must be aesthetic: what can you like and admire?

In these struggles British psychiatrists differ in their views about what their field should include other than schizophrenia, affective psychoses and classical syndromes of neuroses. Dementias, eating disorders, addictions, sexual and marital difficulties, suicidal behaviour, gambling and socially declared perversions, as well as much violence and many personality disorders, often come their way and are often welcomed, despite a lack of agreed psychiatric methods of intervention for them.

The prolonged training and examination system and the professional associations are, however, largely for the professional and marginalize the majority of the population, who are led to believe that they do not know how to treat other people properly, while the professional often believes he does know what he is doing. For the professional any other insight is dangerous. S/he has been socially compliant and academically assiduous in order to achieve the very status that is jeopardized by honest and clear thinking. Would s/he be mad to imperil her/himself? I believe that psychiatrists frequently, at least consistently but often unconsciously, recommend to patients an analogous connivance with socially created realities and call this 'mental health' – unless the pecking order can be altered.[3]

Intelligent psychiatrists see much of the humbug on which their moderately powerful position rests. They are aware that in so many situations Doctor does *not* know best, and they grasp the strangeness of the hierarchical system based on years of training which produces as much status as relevant erudition. The latter can be quickly acquired; but complicity with the *realpolitik* is good, healthy, adjusted commonsense, even if it dehumanizes and debases thought and leaves one wondering what are conversations and case conferences about, even in university departments.

Some psychotic conditions are considered by so many to be such clearly physical conditions that other approaches may only be able to make minor contributions, even if, as we now know, long-term chemical results, at least in schizophrenia, are limited. Psychiatry, however, must also locate itself within other disputes affecting its special relevance to drug addiction, alcoholism, psychopathic personalities, etc., and – despite Freud – psychotherapies. Admit you need help and risk the ready acquiescence of the helpers. Those marginalized by admitting their needs and desires have limited statutory options; but lay, especially self-help, groups are growing up, often hedging their timid bets by accepting psychiatric advisers.

The feeling of being marginalized, though, is relevant to the production of so-called psychiatric conditions. Not surprisingly there is ambivalence about what one should feel about things like being unemployed (especially in a society extolling enterprise) when 'mental health' is a term used to describe those contented with their actual state and possibilities. They are, tautologically, the adjusted. It is assumed that one 'should' in general be happy, want to work, not be frightened, even of dying, be content with one's sex and the clothes it is currently allowed to wear, not want drugs not prescribed by a doctor, and not be paranoid. If you do not feel like this then you have a problem with which a psychiatrist can be approached to cope; s/he will help you to adapt. In addition, s/he is to look after the senile and the simple, or more accurately to tell others

- nurses, home helps, organizers of meals on wheels, wardens and so on - how to help. The fact that at one level of thinking all mental states are cerebral, including, presumably anger, jealousy and mania, makes them all to some extent reducible to brain states, studiable by technologies which cost a great deal and help to make scientists as well as cures. One prong in 'treatment' then is always conceivably pharmacological, even if drug addiction is also a sin and an illness.

Aneurin Bevan and the Labour government established the NHS and bought the medics by 'stuffing them with gold'. Psychiatry was included, after considerable debate, and so psychiatrists were paid as physicians and surgeons. This position as equivalent specialists was very valuable, enhancing the status of mental hospital doctors. They subsequently capitalized on this by establishing a Royal College like those of the older bodies of physicians and surgeons.

However, psychiatry did also become the complex combination of those who ended up in mental hospitals and the discontented, unhappy, hysterical, lonely people Freud claimed to be able to help and to understand. The profession itself, especially in Britain, also became very aware of 'institutional neuroses'[4] - illnesses added by mental hospitals to those the clients brought with them: in fact, apathy and the lack of respect, hope, and individuality.

The current economic climate, including the marginalization of four million unemployed people, gives substance to the Marxist argument that ownership of and the actual means of production produce the person and the psychology of his/her times. Violence in the inner cities, drug addiction, child abuse, football hooliganism, AIDS, big business fraudulence and fear of nuclear war are among the major concerns of modern British society along with the consequences of feminism and the breakdown of the traditional family. These and their consequences are tampered with by psychiatrists seeking their 'proper' niche.

Even if the psychiatrist does not wish to cope with angry and aggressive behaviour, there are many situations in which s/he is pressurized to do so. Cantankerous patients in an old people's home, for example, can be and indeed are pushed her/his way. Where else can they go and who else will be called to general medical or surgical wards to cope with their dissidents?

It is in this context that psychiatry serves to obscure and distance the political and moral dimension and to separate the problems from those of the economic structure. Psychiatry must separate illness from the socioeconomic, or else increase its political ties and decrease its medical links in order to be relevant to the marginalized people it is said to, and does, serve.

Compared to medicine, in psychiatry the agreement on ends is considerably weaker. Yet British psychiatrists prefer technical to moral issues, and as a group are neither overtly political nor asking the central questions about a person's life. For example, the view that schizophrenia has been a product of society since the eighteenth century,[5] on the basis that from that time to be successful in an industrial context has been central, is not provable. Yet it is conceivable that the materialism of scientific industrialization and a liberal faith in progress produced modern man, and that it is relevant to factors affecting the prevalence, presentation and course of schizophrenia, the concept of which it clearly affects. The required marginalization of people who did not fit in led to the asylums too, from which British and other psychiatries grew.

While psychiatrists must be, in limited ways, economists, sociologists and politicians, they are professionals and intellectuals. In order to remain powerful they have been and must be significantly complicit with the status quo, and at least in that sense they must understand the system. British psychiatrists, like those in other countries, have different outlooks but many understandably preach the need to remain physicians. Their science is based on allocation of and ownership of areas of concern and their subsequent history. Those without such property are marginalized.

Separating psychiatric problems from those of life in general clearly marginalizes people. Even therapeutic communities, in which the residents are given the same power as the staff to regulate each other's behaviour, will, if they don't make the whole society become more reflective, produce a subtler police force and control of the marginalized. The government favours a move of psychiatry to the community, but to a leaderless community in which the government's function is only to increase the real police force and prisons and maintain the ring for open and unplanned conflict. The risk to the marginalized will be tranquillizing by drugs, psychotherapy, day hospitals, therapeutic communities, the police, prisons, and the caring of expensive professionals who are experts in controlling. Hence the impending Brave New World, and the complicated, contorted concept of caring.

Currently, British society is becoming also more legalized as well as medicalized. Its morality and marginalizing, however, are very significantly concerned with ownership. To own millions and to improve the techniques of producing and selling coal or newspapers, while devastating the lives of villages and workers, is legal and moral. Damage to property is not. To perpetrate this ideology we must all be encouraged to become shareholders and owners.

This all leads to privatization, and yet legalization, of everything. Perhaps the problems of the elderly illustrate this. Privately 'owned' homes for the elderly (financed by the public sector),[6] for example, have increased by 31 per cent from 1982–4, and to try and assure against abuse we have the Registered Homes Act 1984 and the Health and Social Services and Social Security Adjudication Act. In the UK, 95 per cent of the over 65s live in the community, although the rate of being seriously disabled is more than double in this age group, compared with those under 65. Wenger[7] also shows that dependency needs and domiciliary services are both increasing in the UK, but sadly the former faster than the latter. If correct, what could be more marginalizing? Wenger feels we cannot pursue our intended move to the community without increased resources, which the government thinks should come from private insurance. Wenger also highlights our poor communication between services, GPs, social services departments, social security offices, housing departments, psychiatrists and voluntary agents. This falling between stools, which the lack of integration allows, leads to considerable further marginalization, and makes some case against believing in the ultimate benevolence of market and other blind forces.

Blakemore[8] adds that our fastest growing group is the ageing members of minority racial groups. Local voluntary initiatives predominate in helping these people and statutory services fail to compensate for their well-known reticence to use their provisions. The ethnic minorities raise considerable psychiatric issues, sometimes because of their supposedly 'strange' religions and social practices, especially for their daughters, but primarily because they are not treated equally.

The role played by psychiatry in relation to the elderly has been highlighted for me by the experience I had in Sheffield. To begin with, I was opposed to special services for the elderly, but one evening I was called out to see a 90-year-old man in the casualty department. He was grossly demented. The GP had referred him some months before to an out-patient department which had put him on a waiting list. That morning, however, it was cold and the neighbours had called the doctor because the old man was unclad in his garden, and his house was in disarray without heating and with all the doors open.

The casualty department, however, could not get a psychiatrist to see him. The beds were reported to be full everywhere and they sent him home in an ambulance and asked a social worker to call. The neighbours called the GP, who, now irritated, delivered the man in his own car back to the hospital. There he remained for several hours. Then the bright idea arose that the local professor of psychiatry should be put on his mettle. Reluctantly I admitted him to one of our very precious academic beds, to some extent designated to give some capacity for academic research. I subsequently found that plenty of other beds had been available and of course, with delectable self-righteous indignation, I complained that the university department was being unreasonably coerced.

Two gin and tonics later, the associated hypertension resolved and some critical thought seemed to emerge. The working of the system could be seen in terms of power and status, contradictions and social forces. My colleagues wondered why they should have to take what no-one else wants. They too had interesting things to do; problems which can be largely resolved by good nurses, central heating and food would not support that.

What was in it and for whom, or, more cogently, how could it all be changed? Clearly change could only come by having people in powerful positions who got something out of the services so obviously needed: in other words, psychogeriatricians. We now have four teams of them. I think most of their training is irrelevant because much of what they do can be done, as in the case of the man in question, by untrained people. However, the Royal College of Psychiatrists has a subsection which is represented on all NHS appointments boards to ensure that successful candidates are fully trained and have had adequate experience. This involves some 12 years of training after 'A' levels. Further, the anti-community psychiatry supporters want hospitals, not ho(s)tels.

Nevertheless, the situation in Sheffield has greatly improved. Perhaps one day it will be politically wise to let the old and young interact more freely, not in separate wards and institutions, but using community mental health centres run to a considerable extent by and for those who use them and with much greater flexibility.

For a white, male, Anglo-Saxon professor of psychiatry to write about the marginalized people in Great Britain is almost to refer to nearly everyone else, even if he confesses some damage done to him and his own family by his own ambition. In the short compass of this chapter, it is difficult to do more. I take the neologism, the marginalized, to refer to those whose opinions and needs are referred to only in marginal notes, while the others are considered in the text proper of society's programme. Society must produce cakes as well as cut them up. Productivity needs rewarding, to some extent financially or more subtly by respect, and of course by giving titles – knighthoods, professorships, Doctor, Senior Principal Chief this and that. Much dissidence is obviated when an individual is doing his third year for the OBE. Complicit involvement in social structures is also a large aspect of almost everyone's life. It involves accepting the pecking order, being polite, speaking the language which opens the door, and it involves indifference to the marginalized.

Psychiatry tends to marginalize, or at least to confirm marginalization, by its struggle to concretize and objectify its classification system as well as by exaggerating its expertise. Then the individual with certain problems and experiences is schizophrenic, and the losers in interpersonal struggles become patients, with experts agreeing to that and even getting them off legal charges for otherwise immoral behaviour. In the same way as the science of physics extracts ideal cases (for example, perfect gases, frictionless slopes) so that mathematical calculations can lead to useful real applications, psychiatry's would-be medical scientists produce concepts of diseases which statistically can allow one to predict, control and treat. However, that makes the subject an object of science, and so psychiatry is happily made an objective study. It also makes the scientist powerful in his interaction with the patient. Perhaps the paradigms of positivistic science are most out of place when issues are political; in psychiatry they are often at the level of personal politics. The expert risks marginalizing by confirming or denying the issues of such politics. Knowledge, even pseudo-knowledge, is power, and significantly produced to control when caring is more valid.

The psychiatric services in Britain are also splintering into all sorts of subspecialities: mental handicap, forensic psychiatry, biological psychiatry, psychotherapy, drug addiction, psychogeriatrics, child psychiatry, adolescent psychiatry, family psychiatry, social psychiatry, and marital and sexual psychiatry. Each of these is pretending that a great deal of experience and learning is required and many are joining the great educational scandal which succeeds in disenfranchising those without its usually fairly irrelevant diplomas. At the same time, some sort of battle or modus vivendi with non-medical specialists playing the same sorts of games is in progress. They are the nurses, psychologists, lay therapists, social workers, occupational therapists, art therapists, behaviour therapists and hypnotists, all spreading multiple diplomatosis.

This army, with the police and others, are living on the problems of that smallish group of marginalized people who can be called mental patients. Psychiatry and that group both have their origins in the same sociohistoric processes.

Psychiatrists are comparatively wealthy and they have a problem that, if mental illness is defined restrictively, it limits them; if defined widely, it overwhelms them and they cannot maintain their hegemony. The psychiatrist has traditionally been a team leader, which s/he naturally resists relinquishing. S/he still wields more power than the other professionals, and s/he has a special expertise, the use of drug therapies, of which there are essentially only about six types. The move towards real teamwork is obviously progressing in Britain, despite vested interests impeding it. Reactionaries and radicals have to succumb to reason and, if skilled, accept what cannot be respectably defended, while working away to re-establish what they want and can salvage by some other means. As in the problem of hysteria versus malingering, the degree of conscious complicity is imponderable.

For many of the problems, home helps are more useful than psychogeriatricians; a personal welcome to the theatre, rock climbing, pot-holing, a place in a commune, or an ordinary home, camping, music, dancing, painting, each with other ordinary people, is better than psychoanalysis; and certainly jobs would help many. Unfortunately, the structures significantly compete with such flexibility and the structures are by definition only marginally designed for the marginalized.

References

1. Marx and Engels (1845).
2. Marx (1844) *Economic and Philosophical Manuscripts*.
3. Here there is not enough space to present the case for considering schizophrenia and other psychiatric states as significantly reluctance or inability to collude (see, however, for such an attempt, Jenner, F.A. (1984) 'Beyond Complicity and Schizophrenia', *Journal of the British Association of Art Therapists*, Winter, pp. 3-6.
4. Burton, R. (1959) *Institutional Neurosis*, Wright, Bristol.
5. Toney, E.F. (1980) *Schizophrenia and Civilization*, Jason Aronson, Ottawa.
6. Day, P. (1985) 'Regulating the Private Sector of Welfare', *The Political Quarterly*, 56, pp. 282-5.
7. Wenger, G.C. (1985) 'Care in the Community', *Ageing and Society*, 5, pp. 143-59.
8. Blakemore, K. (1985) 'The State, Voluntary Sector and New Developments in Provision for the Old and Minority Racial Groups', *Ageing and Society*, 5, pp. 175-90.

10

Treating Social Marginality in the South of Italy

ROCCO CANOSA

When Pinel – influenced by the logic of the Enlightenment and inspired by the libertarian examples of the French Revolution – frees the insane from the chains which kept them confused with criminality, then he in fact begins to separate out the world of misery and unreason by giving madness a different qualitative connotation. All of this causes the fragmentation of more urgent global demands from the masses and the structuring of a new logic which facilitates their evasion by setting up technical responses of which psychiatry is one example[1] ... Conferring a sort of scientific dignity on unreason means avoiding replying to what expresses itself in its own language: oppression, poverty, want. Middle-class rationale has kept hunger and poverty in the necessary compartments for balancing the economic logic upon which it is based but has produced the impoverishment of human existence within its own breast.[2]

By working on the relationship between misery and power it has been possible to produce practices which have led to the superseding of the mental hospital and to the new law on psychiatric welfare in Italy.

In the transition from the institutionalized totality of the mental hospital to the decentralized institution of the neighbourhood area, the psychiatric services have been entrusted with problems which were relatively unknown to them before the new law. These vary from the young unemployed with psychological problems and children with difficulties in school to the old and lonely and to those in prison. At the same time the agencies designated for control of these groups of 'marginals' (for example, the justice system, the police, the social services) tend to delegate responsibility for them to the psychiatric services. All this has been happening when alongside successive cuts in health and welfare expenditure a review of institutional thinking and practice has been taking place: youth institutes have been transformed into apartment groups, mental hospitals converted back into rehabilitation units, old people's homes repainted and cleaned and communities for drug dependents have been created.

It is interesting to note how the tendency for institutions to delegate a series of problems which are on the boundaries of psychiatry to the psychiatric services has produced in Italy two very different lines of approach for mental health workers. The first is to consider problems which are not exclusively clinical to be 'rejects' from psychiatry and therefore within the scope of the social services. The other arises from thinking of treatment as 'being responsible for someone', as looking after the person in the complexity of his/her requirements. From this, it is not necessary to fragment the vast richness of personal situations according to area of professional competence, but to consider them instead as unique conditions so that the encounter between user and worker may take place subjectively and outside the scope of any trite technical means.

By situating themselves at the crossroads of health and welfare and by taking the responsibility for marginal cases, these services are in fact playing a supporting role to ineffective or inefficient structures and services. Italy, which in the past has only partially moved towards being a welfare state, is currently experiencing an economic and ideological crisis, alongside many Western countries. As a result of this, many social health services are declining or disappearing altogether. Most psychiatric users, if directed exclusively to the social services for problems not strictly clinical, would now more than ever before risk total neglect.

The problem of resources in the mental health service has therefore become central. The service, which aims to resist increasing attempts to abandon the weakest to 'their fate', needs resources not only for financial benefits, but also canteens, holidays, workers' co-operatives, training programmes, outings and celebrations, the provision of comfortable meeting places and an adequate number of staff.

The worker/user relationship has also been altered and has assumed 'therapeutic transparency' through the use of the resources available and the concreteness of the responses, which include financial benefits. Firstly this enabled us to attempt the restoration of the internal suffering of the individual's overall existence to the inside of his or her own identity; a process of reappropriation. Secondly, the use of environmental resources has been the means by which the therapeutic relationship has been revealed as one of dependence, power and dispossession. Finally the use of resources has shaped the user's social awareness.[3]

For example, think how many emotional factors come into play during a seaside stay, and how many opportunities may arise for a remarkable change in the traditional relationship between carer and patient. It must be emphasized that this experience of being together is not something outside ordinary therapy (whether it be psychological or pharmaceutical); but it is not about occupational therapy. It is an integral part of the total therapeutic relationship, articulated in its complexity, sometimes difficult, often contradictory, but involving workers beyond their roles and specialisms. The user's needs are not divided into medicinal, psychological, monetary and so on, nor do individual specialist workers correspond to each type of need. What is attempted is recognition of all the user's problems in order to be able to respond to them globally.

This type of relationship also has profound implications for how work is organized. It must be flexible not bureaucratic; be able to adapt to changing demands. It should be aimed at using individual professions within a complex programme of treatment, by establishing collective objectives of change in the everyday practice of both users and the service/institution.

To give an example of this type of work it would be useful to outline the experience of the Bari San Paolo Mental Health Service in Puglia, beginning with information on the relevant welfare and socioeconomic context.

The Socioeconomic Profile of Puglia

Puglia, a region in southern Italy, has 3,871,617 inhabitants with an 8.4 per cent population increase in the last decade. Between 1979 and 1983 agricultural employment declined by 17.2 per cent, industrial employment increased slightly by 0.6 per cent and there was a 12.1 per cent increase in the service sector.

Between 1981 and 1983 unemployment has increased from 8.4 per cent to 11.2 per cent. Annual per capita income in Puglia[4] is lower than both the average for southern regions and the national average. Housing shortage is high(1981 census). The number of eviction procedures which took place in just the first quarter of 1983 represents 10.1 per cent of the national total. These data provide crude evidence that income, work and housing are lacking in Puglia.

Psychiatry in Puglia

Psychiatric welfare in Puglia has been dominated by the presence of three large psychiatric hospitals: Bisceglie (BA) and Foggia which are privately owned by a religious organization (*Case Della Divina*

Provvidenza) and the psychiatric hospital in Lecce which is publicly owned. In the face of this massive private institutional presence, private neuropsychiatric clinics have had little place and in Puglia there are only three (two at Bari and one at Lecce) with few beds. The university clinic (with 72 beds), which before the introduction of Law 180 functioned first as a channel of referral and then as a filter of patients to the psychiatric hospital, has become the local psychiatric unit in the general hospital. During the 1970s the number of patients in the three psychiatric hospitals in Puglia stayed almost constant, varying between 4,468 and 4,934. Between 1979 and 1983 the numbers of patients declined from 3,964 to 3,060. During this period the number of patients in Bisceglie hospital declined by 26.6 per cent (with 16.9 per cent dying); in Lecce by 27.2 per cent (of whom 11.1 per cent died), while in Foggia's hospital the situation remained unchanged. Overall, only 6.8 per cent of patients were discharged from the psychiatric hospitals in Puglia.[5]

Concerning compulsory treatment carried out by the psychiatric wards in general hospitals there was a decline of 26 per cent from 905 in 1979 to 669 in 1983.[6] During the two years 1980–81, 1,621 proposals for compulsory treatment were put forward in the province of Bari, but the district psychiatric services approved only 427.[7] In 1981 the number of new users of all the district services in the region was 2,314; in 1983 this figure was 10,896.[8] The number of employees in these services is 60 per cent less than the number forecast in the process of planning.

The psychiatric hospitals resisted the discharging of patients. This can be understood if it is noted that the psychiatric hospitals at Bisceglie and Foggia received as a rule more than 70 billion lire annually for patients from public sources. If these were discharged the earnings would diminish. In addition, private psychiatric hospitals as well as the public one at Lecce have tended to convert themselves into rehabilitation institutions in order to ensure their survival; proposals to this end have already been submitted to the regional authorities.

Despite the great lack of resources, the new psychiatric services have succeeded in filtering requests for admissions, which are no longer passed through the old segregating channels, and in taking charge of greatly increased numbers of new users.

The Mental Health Service at San Paolo, Bari

The experience of the mental health service at San Paolo, Bari took place within this framework: San Paolo is a district of Bari with more than 50,000 inhabitants, situated 10km from the city centre. Built 20 years ago to provide a refuge for people from the old city and suburban hovels, it has one of the highest rates of juvenile delinquency in Italy and very high rates of truancy and unemployment.[9] It is the expression of a kind of 'mental hospital mentality', since like a mental hospital it is isolated from the rest of the city; it contains the unproductive and deviant social groupings; and it is where violence, squalor and deprivation are the norm.

Work in the District

A group of psychiatric workers chose to work in this district where the schools are inadequate, sanitation services lacking and social services practically non-existent. In the initial stage (October 1981) the team was made up of only one doctor, two social workers and three nurses, with accommodation on the premises of the service for old people. This choice was made to avoid certain disadvantages to the users who had been obliged to attend a distant service in the centre of Bari, and to avoid continuing a service which had in fact been limited to sporadic consultations and emergency stop-gap measures and which was then significantly inferior to treatment offered in the Bisceglie mental hospital and the university clinic.

An immediate change was experienced in the quality of the relationship with the users and their families: a rigid and bureaucratic relationship became more direct and lively. The people of the district could hardly believe that it was no longer necessary to queue interminably in order to obtain a consultation; that rubber-stamping was no longer necessary for health service; that a free public service was able to provide a whole team for home consultations.

In addition, increasing numbers of the young unemployed, young women weary from constantly and haphazardly tending their numerous children, pensioners requiring medicine, and ex-prisoners out of work began using the service along with people with severe psychic disorders and with histories of violence and poverty. We asked ourselves: where was psychiatry as we had been taught to recognize it? It was dramatically present in the serious individual disorders but the various forms of widespread deprivation were not taken into consideration.

We realized that we could not remain locked in our specific service and we sought to liaise with the other health and social services who had similar problems to ours in terms of scarce resources.

In the spring of 1982 a co-ordinating committee of the service workers was created. It produced an analysis and specific proposals for improving the quality of the service. The co-ordinating body also took part in the activities of the district's 'Committee for the Struggle for

Social Services' which had also been created and which initiated a dispute with the Bari local authority on a whole series of unresolved problems (from the schools to the road network, the water system and transportation facilities). This mobilization produced some important results (for instance, the allocation of 3 billion lire for the infrastructure). Above all, by means of the collective momentum of confrontation and struggle it contributed to the beginnings of a slow reconstruction of something which had been brutally destroyed in the people of San Paolo: a sense of solidarity.

At Bisceglie Mental Hospital

During the Spring and Summer of 1982, while the work in the district was being carried out, the nurses who had been transferred from Bisceglie hospital started to contact within the mental hospital patients who came originally from their catchment area. This work was not merely another activity of the district work, because of the weight of that psychiatric institution. The latter was used by society to screen out the reality which had to remain invisible.[10]

The knowledge that no district psychiatric service could be effective or efficient if it existed alongside the mental hospital rather than *as an alternative* to it was based on this analysis. Progress was made from the regular consultations which workers used to have with the psychiatric hospital patients to the first outings in the city, tours and a stay in a seaside hotel (Summer 1982).

These initiatives were taken in the belief that reintroducing people into society who had been confined to a mental hospital for decades would be a gradual process. This would also require new resources if more deprivation and neglect were to be avoided. The seaside holiday in particular demonstrated the enormous capacity of the patients for reappropriating their space and privacy much more quickly than had been expected and which even many years in the hospital had not succeeded in destroying.

During the following years the relationship with these patients developed; rehabilitation work continued and many of them were finally discharged. The following two examples are provided as illustration of the style of work of the service.

F., a young man of 23, is diagnosed as having 'schizophrenia with mental handicap'. This was the outcome of a psychotic episode which he had at the age of eight. He was always misbehaving, with some aggression; was hospitalized many times on a compulsory basis or stayed in prison because of burglaries committed with others.

Initially, the service has attempted to talk with him (he used only few and incomprehensible phrases), to offer him a space to come and stay as he wished, to manage his financial benefits for him, enable him to participate in outings, help him in sorting out physical ill health (like going with him to the dentist and GP), encourage and arrange for him to go back to school, to meet his family, helping the latter to recognize his achievements. The results are very positive: for many months now he has not been hospitalized, had no brushes with the law. He is listened to by others who do not consider him any more to be incurably 'mad' or 'stupid'.

The second example concerns a 50-year-old woman who had been in the psychiatric hospital for 30 years for 'acute psychosis'. We met her for the first time four years ago. She was dressed in a long skirt of a nondescript blue, always in a corner, never said a word and was incontinent. On her clinical file she was described as 'demented schizophrenic'. When we asked her to join us for vacation, the hospital nurses smiled ironically saying, 'It is all useless; can't you see that she is incurable?'

In the beginning we taught her to use knives and forks while eating (the hospital allows only the use of a spoon), to dress and wash herself. We sat for long periods with her, talking endlessly, attempting to understand her gestures, looks, her hardly recognizable smiles, sudden flashes of fury and her wish to start again after so many lost years. For the last two years she has lived in a group home with other severe ex-patients. She can now cook, and helps with domestic tasks. At times she speaks a lot about herself, sings old songs and often smiles gently.

The relatively new mental health service in San Paolo has demonstrated in its activities and record that it is possible to offer a psychiatric service focused on the totality of the individual and not on his/her psychiatric symptomatology. This approach means that people viewed as marginals of any type are referred and refer themselves to this kind of service. This has been achieved despite the very deprived conditions of the area, the hostile administration and the scandalous continued existence of the private psychiatric hospital which thrives on public funds. It has been achieved because of its workers' commitment to become part of and use the area's social resources.

References

1. Basaglia, F. Ongaro (1981) *Introduzione in Inventario di una psichiatria*, Electa, Milan.
2. Ibid.
3. Gallio G., Giannichedda M.G., De Leonardis O., Mauri, D. (1983) *La*

Libertà è Terapeutica? L'esperienza psichiatrica di Trieste, Feltrinelli, Milan.

4. Dati ISTAT (1984) on the Puglia region.
5. *Osservatorio di Epidemiologia Servizio Igiene Mentale di Bari* (1984) *Dati sull'assistenza psichiatrica in Puglia*, Bari.
6. Ibid.
7. Ibid.
8. Ibid.
9. Ibid.
10. Maccacaro, G.A. (1975) 'Ipotesi di ricerca, programma finalizzato', *Medicina Preventiva*, subprogetto Prevenzione Malattie Mentali, C.N.R., Rome.

11

Defining and Experimenting with Prevention

SUE HOLLAND

This is an opportune time to write on the subject of prevention with the publication of MIND's 'Charter 2000 Action Programmes for a World in Crisis'.[1] The charter's section on 'prevention of mental illness/promotion of mental health' makes a rhetorical plea to governments and public authorities to

> endeavour to maintain basic social stability, harmonious relationships between social/cultural groups and reduce stigma and discrimination associated with different racial, sexual or religious groupings, [also, to] ensure that the environment is as conducive as possible to mental health.

Unfortunately the charter does not suggest what is to be done if 'government(s)' choose not to respond along these progressive lines. The charter has apparently overlooked the fact that, in Britain at least, 'governments' have been moving quite firmly in the opposite direction. Structural factors which are now known to increase the risk of pushing people towards and over the brink of mental breakdown, such as unemployment, poverty, racism, unsafe and stressful working conditions, homelessness and bad housing, are all on the increase. For example, Brown and Harris's[2] findings reported in *Social Origins of Depression* that the lack of nursery places and jobs for women could contribute towards women's vulnerability to depression were not followed by governmental policies for creation of nursery places and jobs for women, but the very opposite. MIND in its prestigious world conferences and charters continues to ignore the discrepancy between the apparent influence on mental health of destructive social conditions and the state's structural inability to respond humanely. The question is not whether mental illness *could* be prevented – there is now sufficient indication that much of the emotional and social dis-ease and distress known as mental illness could be prevented – but *who* wants to prevent it? The medico-psychiatric professions have shown scant interest in questions of prevention. For example, a library search of index medicus (after 1980) on depressive disorder (the most prevalent mental illness) produced approximately 7,000 articles, but only three on depressive disorder and primary prevention (none of them British).

It can be argued that at both the personal unconscious level of the sufferer or 'patient' and the public structural level of the state, there is a conspiracy of silence to maintain the condition of 'madness'; the former as a protection against the stark truth of his/her social existence, the latter as a manifestation of its power and control. This leads to the core assumption of this chapter: that the issue of mental illness is both profoundly subjective and profoundly political. Prevention must therefore be addressed to both the internalized social structures (object relations) of the human psyche and the external social structures (class, gender, race) of society and state. The prescriptions for 'treatment' which follow from such a model include both psychotherapeutic intervention at the psychic level, and political action at the structural level. It is not a model readily found within the British welfare system of psychiatry or other mental health professions.

Preventing What and in Whose Communities?

Within the present British psychiatric services there is some agreement, at least within the medico-psychiatric professional establishment, as to what is mental illness, but apparently little agreement as to what *causes* it. Consequently, there is no general agreement as to what measures must be taken to *prevent* it. In fact, all aspects related to the aetiology, treatment and prevention of diagnosed mental illness is riven with controversy; as readily admitted by the newer psychiatric establishment (see Anthony Clare's *Psychiatry in Dissent*).[3] Three areas of prevention are recognized, primary, secondary and tertiary, but psychiatry pays little attention to the first, concentrating instead on the secondary 'nipping-in-the-bud' of acute mental breakdown and the tertiary rehabilitation of chronically institutionalized mental hospital patients.

The present government policy of closure of the large old psychiatric hospitals has split the 'psy' professions into opposing camps. Advocates of the community mental health centre (CMHC) welcome the closures and see the community as the proper arena for both prevention and rehabilitation. The old guard in the psychiatric hospitals express doubts as to the readiness of the community to receive its socially vulnerable inmates (who are not only institutionalized but possibly irreversibly brain-damaged by chemico-physical 'treatments'). Each side in the argument has professional territory to hold or to win (see the recent British Psychological Society correspondence between the psychiatrist, Weller, and the psychologist, Pilgrim, regarding the proposed closure of Friern hospital).[4]

The move from psychiatric hospital to the community was given its first ministerial direction in 1961. The policy has elements of both progressive reform and reactionary opportunism, and an avaricious eye for the real estate values of the land on which stand the old work house-cum-asylum-cum-psychiatric hospitals. The proposal is that the chronically incarcerated inmates would be released (decarcerated) into the caring and, hopefully, less expensive 'community' (in actuality, women relatives or landladies). The funding which would help to prepare the community for this caring role has not yet materialized, nor has the original ideal of the CMHC as the focus for prevention and positive mental health. By the mid-1970s a few places calling themselves Community Mental Health, Mental Health Advice, or Crisis Intervention Service Centres had opened with the support of the local authorities: Brindle House in Thameside, Handen Road in Lewisham and the Crisis Intervention Service in Tower Hamlets are well publicized examples. These are, in the British context, experimental, innovative and progressive but all have adopted the orthodox medico-psychiatric model in which a consultant psychiatrist has overall clinical authority, albeit a liberal one (see Goldie[5] for nuances of power in such a model). By the 1980s the now well established model of the CMHC forms the stepping stone onto which psychiatry has made its territorial move out of the hospital and into the community.[6] To do this, it has had to adopt the language of social causal models such as 'psycho-social transitions' or 'life-events'. But in spite of this, none of the issues concerning the effects on mental health of the environment, work, housing, poverty, racism, sexism, ageism, are considered to be appropriate subjects for preventive action. The white coat has been shed for Fair Isle sweaters and chukka boots but the old individualistic organic model of treatment still remains: prescriptions for tranquillizers, anti-depressants, and a community psychiatric nurse (CPN) to drop by with an injection of Depixol, are now accompanied by 'psycho-social counselling'.

Hospitalization of the Community

The proliferation of CMHCs has been divorced from the demands of the people of that community for social change. The recognition of the psyche and the social in mental health has imperceptibly merged with the psy-orientation which endlessly administers to the mentally ill, who, like the poor, are always with us. Structural issues concerning power, wealth and domination and the ideology which helps maintain such a system is never taken as the context in which mental health/illness is socially constructed, but merely as the backdrop to which individual and family dramas are enacted. Psychiatry, by bringing its 'eclectic' baggage of psycho-social language and pharmacological treatments with it into the community, has contributed, not to the communalization of the patient, but to the hospitalization of the community. This has gone alongside developments within other sectors of state welfarism, primary health care and voluntary work. The radical movements of the 1960s for mental health through personal protest and collective action have already been pre-empted, incorporated, and neutralized as 'self-help' and 'community care', a euphemism for the underprivileged to take care of themselves on the cheap. The Dutch radicals in the mental health field have been more alert to this pervasive co-option. A 1983 congress in Utrecht describes the process:

> With the extension of the welfare state the mental health care has become part of the care-complex, which meets all the individual and group problems and also assists in trying to solve these problems. The principle of participation has become a feature of the care-complex, especially from the beginning of the sixties. This participation idea has been worked out in the mental health care only later on. Participation appears in the following form: self-help and mantle-help; with this an informal care-system is created, in which persons are 'made' responsible for themselves and for others. A part of the service is therefore pushed off to this informal sector – this has the consequence that many problems are transferred to women in a predominantly patriarchal world.[7]

It is in this historical context of the ongoing struggle between forces for progressive emancipation and reactionary co-option that the author's two attempts toward prevention are now described: the first a voluntary grant-aided mental health centre, the second a central government funded social services project for depressed women.

Innovation and Co-option

The model of mental health in which preventive work is carried out within the dual context of individual psychotherapeutic change and collective social action is a relatively rare phenomenon within the British mental health scene. The People's Aid and Action Centre started in 1972 and later renamed the Battersea Action and Counselling Centre was the first of its kind.[8] The centre originated out of the collective efforts of a group of community activists, the Wandsworth Community Workshop, which included professional mental health workers. It was situated in a shop-front on a high street, and provided a skilled psychotherapy/counselling service, a day nursery for under-fives, and a greengrocers for pensioners and the unemployed. The main aim of the centre was to help people with personal and material problems, and to increase knowledge and understanding of mental health issues. The kinds of problems included severe depression, marital conflicts, difficulties with children, and general stress and irritability with everyday pressures. The centre's staff played an important role, in partnership with the Wandsworth and East Merton Community Health Council, in helping a group of council tenants to collect the relevant psychosocial evidence in order to demand a transfer from a high-rise block of flats. Making the conceptual link between reflective personal insight and combative social action was a real option for people using the centre in its early days when community action and tenants' struggles were at a peak. Later, as these grassroots organizations became more formalized and co-opted into the fabric of urban local estate management,[9] the centre was thrown back on itself to initiate the kind of structures and resources which its original mental health aims demanded.

Two initiatives made by local users of the centre could have grown into more robust social structures; these were the greengrocers set up by a disabled pensioner, and the nursery which was run by mothers who had originally come to the centre complaining of depression. For various reasons, partly economic, partly idiosyncratic, they did not. Instead, by its fifth year many of the centre's user-participants had been replaced by an influx of educationally privileged radicals who were attracted by its progressive and alternative approach to mental health but who had no involvement with the local working-class community. The centre's failure to initiate the social networks necessary to achieve its social–psychotherapeutic aims led to its withdrawal into more individual forms of therapy whilst at the same time mounting an active educational campaign with people other than its own 'clients'. This led to the usual split between an underprivileged clientele and an educationally sophisticated staff. When the project's funds were withdrawn by the borough's incoming Tory administration of 1979, these radicals found themselves to be the new experts in the now fashionable field of community mental health. They used their experience at the centre to further their careers as mental health consultants, lecturers, and feminist psychotherapists. This failure to engage the working-class users in a way which would invest them with authority and identification with the centre meant there was no strong commitment to the centre from within the working-class community when the grant was withdrawn, and the centre closed its doors. Also, the neighbourhood had become 'gentrified' as private tenants moved out of the now fashionable and expensive terraced houses 'a stone's throw from Chelsea Bridge'. It was no surprise when the centre's vacant premises reopened as a cocktail bar. Some of those radicals who had been involved with the centre later published articles to try to account for the difficulty experienced in helping working-class people to articulate that 'unhappy silence' which was their mental distress: 'There was a huge need for the kind of intervention we wished to make but we were surprised by the apparent lack of demand for it once we became established.'[10]

Having failed in practice to engage with this 'unhappy silence', and having lost their physical base within the neighbourhood, they regrouped in Lambeth in the form more familiar to them; the discussion workshop. From here they reiterated in an alternative 'discourse' what had been said already but now published for a wider professional audience:

> This is the arena where the most forceful encounter occurs between the discourses of the ideological subject and of the subject of the unconscious; ... it allows consideration of both social and psychoanalytic subjectification; put more simply, it deals with the intertwined realities of private and public experience.[11]

One crucial problem faced by the centre was that ideally, funds should have been available to pay local volunteers who wanted to be involved in the work of the centre but who were neither privileged nor eccentric enough to do it for nothing. Unfortunately, such an arrangement went against both the prevailing trend for recruiting unpaid 'good neighbours' and the trade unions' understandably defensive hostility to volunteer programmes. Neither view lent itself to supporting the development of a genuinely participatory and collective approach to mutual care within the neighbourhood.

Service and Transformation

The lesson learned here was that any new venture in the field of preventive work in mental health must make as its central task the transformation of passive receivers of mental health services into active participants in the understanding and the solutions to their own and their neighbours' mental distress. Paradoxically, this task has been more nearly accomplished within the less radically ambitious and more orthodox setting of the social services project. The scheme, started in October 1980 by Hammersmith and Fulham Social Services and funded by the Department of the Environment, has the four-tiered approach of intensive focal psychotherapy, group work, mental health education and the stimulation of mutual-help initiatives within the neighbourhood. The client group are women and their families on a housing estate, who are considered to be vulnerable to depressive breakdown. The model for intervention was created utilizing skills and methods developed both through the author's psychodynamic training at the Tavistock Clinic and the years of community practice engaged in during the Battersea project. From these strands of influence was created a theory and practice which attempted to grasp the dialectic of psychic world (inside) and social structure (outside). The steps in this therapeutic practice, or 'social action psychotherapy' are: Symptom into Knowledge (insight) into Desire into Action.

The stages of this intervention can be placed within a theoretical framework provided by Burrell and Morgan's Four Paradigms for the Analysis of Social Theory and which has been developed into a radical method of teaching social theory to social work students by Colin Whittington and Ray Holland.[12] This theoretical framework proposes two dimensions: Radical change – Regulation; Subjective – Objective; which represents vertical and horizontal axes in relation to which social theories can be located. The four sectors produced by these intersecting dimensions are the four key paradigms: Functionalist, Interpretive, Radical Humanist and Radical Structuralist. This theoretical model has proved useful in trying to convey the quality of the changes involved in therapy which aims to move the depressed woman from individual Symptom, into Psychic Knowledge, into shared Desire into Social Action – (see diagram and explanatory note).

Parameters of Change

	Radical	Radical	
	Humanism	Structuralism	
	Shared	Social	
	Desire	**Action**	

Subjective   Objective

Psychic Individual

| | **Meaning** | **Symptom** |
| | Interpretive | Functionalism |

Regulation

The horizontal dimension runs between the objective and subjective poles. *Objectivism* emphasizes a natural science model; the organism, or even the machine. Things are measured and quantified. The other polar extreme is *subjectivism* which emphasizes the unique qualities of human experience, interpretation of meanings and use of symbols. The vertical dimension at one end suggests a relatively static or slowly evolving social situation, and the other one in which radical change is an inevitable, even desirable state. (Adapted from Burrell and Morgan).[13]

Although the work aims to intervene before serious depressive breakdown is reached, in fact, due to the long history of superficial and pharmacological response to women's depression on this estate by the medical services, much of the work is with women who have gone through repeated episodes of crippling depression, sometimes resulting in hospitalization. Typical are the women who went to their GP eight or ten years ago following a bereavement or separation and who have now become dependent on the sleeping pills and tranquillizers they were offered to suppress their grief, agitation and anger.

Such women originally presented themselves at the GP's using the functionalist language which they had learned was the correct way to describe their discomfort to a doctor, that is as symptoms ... 'my nerves'. Starting with the depressed woman who sees her problems in functionalist terms, the programmes of therapy offered in the project aim to move her through into the interpretive mode or paradigm: 'What does your depression mean and where does it come from?' Then, by way of group work into the radical humanist mode: 'What do you want of yourself and others?' Finally, and this is the most difficult, into the radical structuralist mode: 'What is to be done?' 'How can we change the bit of the world we inhabit?' This is the problem of action, both individual and collective.

Movement through the different modes or paradigms is achieved by providing intensive individual therapy which focuses on key issues and which is time limited to a period of a few months. The woman then moves into educational and conscientization groups (the term coined by Freire[14] is preferred as it incorporates the element of collective history and cultural awareness). The educational groups aim to locate women's mental health within the context of family and society. One of the conscientization groups has brought together women from different ethnic and national backgrounds to discuss the issues, contradictions, pleasures and pains of being in 'mixed' marriages. For example, the unconscious racialism which may lurk beneath the white woman's sexual feelings for her black partner and which is given fuel by the openly racist structures within the state.[15] Another group, the Afro-Caribbean Women's History Group, has brought together black women who have known severe depression and who now want to relate their personal suffering to the wider context of their collective history and present life in Britain.

In this project there was no built-in proposal for how the fourth mode be achieved, it being more appropriate that this would grow out of the previous modes. After three years this materialized as a core group of women, using the groups to help build their confidence and knowledge, who formed a separate project, Women's Action for Mental Health, with its own grant from the GLC (Greater London Council) Women's Committee. Through the project they provide a neighbourhood counselling and general support, advice and activities service with two co-ordinators/counsellors, a book-keeper/administrator, a cleaner and two creche workers (all providing very well paid jobs for local women). It has been this development which has taken the women into the fourth mode in which they have changed things within their environment and raised the question of mental health as a social issue within their housing estate. It has also involved them in the local politics of housing allocation as their need for premises was at first blocked by the housing chairman. This escalated into the illegal occupation of the desired premises by the women, who were then labelled 'criminals' by the said councillor (see Sarah Caldwell's article in the *Guardian*, 25 May 1984). The social services directorate were now embarrassed that this had become a 'political issue', revealing that the central contradiction is that statutory welfare agencies which promote 'self-help' models of mental health care cannot tolerate it when oppressed patient/clients *do* help themselves and each other.[16]

In contrast to the newly gentrified Battersea of the 1970s, this Hammersmith estate of the 1980s is seen as the end-of-the-line for people who have failed to find anywhere better: the homeless, displaced immigrants, unemployed, single mothers, black and ethnic minority people, as well as the original English families who first moved in when the estate was a 'showcase' for the white working classes.

The women shared a common anger that they as residents were personally stigmatized because of the public failure of housing policy over the decades. By making demands as to how a particular building on the estate should be used, they were throwing off the perception of themselves as passive victims of that housing policy. They gained so much public support from tenants, professionals, voluntary workers, councillors, and the church, that their demands were met and they were given tenancy of the premises.

The reason the women got so much neighbourhood support was that they were locals themselves and had a network of neighbours, relatives and friends who they persuaded with their own enthusiasm and belief in what they were doing. In spite of the popular prejudice for anything involving the word 'mental' they were able to persuade a large number of residents on the estate that the mental health of women and their families was a matter for neighbourhood concern and public interest. They quickly learnt how to engage the local press and how to find their way around the council bureaucracy; achievements which enhanced their self-esteem and feelings of competence.

From Personal Symptom to Political Action

This progression within a neighbourhood therapy programme could be described in terms of trying to move the depressed woman through psychic space into social space and so into political space. This is precisely the point at which neurotic symptoms or hostility towards the internalized failed or lost object/person should be disengaged from the just rage felt towards oppression in the outside world. Psychic space is not the same as political space, but the former can sabotage the person's struggle with the latter.[17]

It is from this arena of struggle with the *outside* world that the mentally ill person has run away, and it is an arena in which there are real rather than imagined enemies (not a fashionable idea amongst the 'psy' professions at present who have retreated into self-satisfied pacifism).[18] The question for prevention, as in psychotherapy, is the question of who and what is *preventing* change in a progressive and humane direction? Only those who are the present victims of the prevailing destructive social conditions will have a true commitment to the struggle towards prevention. It is also they who will be the main recipients of the British welfare state's attempt to treat, administer, therapeutize, tranquillize and neutralize them out of their justifiable rage.

Working-class housing estates and neighbourhoods are used as the 'hospital' outside the walls of the hospital. The old psychiatric diagnosis and passive receipt of treatment by the patient are likely to continue to be the cornerstone of the 'new' community mental health resource centres of the late 1980s. Alternatively, definitions of and solutions to mental-health-at-risk should arise from the members of a community itself. We do not have as yet examples of a British community taking this stance in regard to questions of mental health. The forces working against members of a community defining their own mental health needs are massive; the ideological influence of a class system rooted in deference, individualism and awesome respect for medical experts militates against such a move. Recently there have been stirrings coming from sectors within the black and ethnic minority communities (professional and lay, statutory and voluntary) and the women's movement (see the work of the Ethnic Studies Group, Nafsiyat, Islington Women and Mental Health and the Women's Therapy Centre).

Community and advice centres which serve black and ethnic minority people are now turning their attention to the question of mental health out of a sheer necessity to protect their clients from a psychiatric system which processes them without understanding or sympathy. Black youth and their parents are now beginning to question the reason why so many of them are arrested on the streets and compulsorily hospitalized under section 136 of the 1983 Mental Health Act. From all these sectors there is a growing criticism of the 'psy' professions' duplicity with the welfare state in reducing public oppression to matters of private psychic despair. However well meaning and identified with the oppressed the mental health professionals are, our attempts to help will always be sabotaged by the recipients' humiliation and resentment at having to need help. It is only by finding a therapeutic practice which will genuinely empower the 'patient/client' that we can honestly reject the accusation that we are 'poverty-pimps' enriching ourselves out of the anguish of others.

A preventative programme for mental-health-at-risk would engage those sectors of the population, including working-class women, black, Irish and Asian minority people, redundant working men and the unemployed youth of all these groups. It would offer an alternative model of personal change, social-consciousness-raising and collective action. The measure of its success will be a new-born confidence amongst the recipients of these methods, to question the routes both personal and social by which they arrived at definitions of themselves and their neighbours as mentally ill. The conclusions for future action which they will draw from this are yet unknown but will be the truly new territory for preventive schemes in mental health.

References

1. Charter 2000 (1985) *Brighton Declarations on the Rights of Mentally Ill People and the Promotion of Mental Health*, MIND.
2. Brown, G., Harris, T. (1978) *Social Origins of Depression*, Tavistock, London.
3. Clare, A. (1978) *Psychiatry in Dissent*, Tavistock, London.
4. BPS correspondence: Pilgrim, D., Weller, M. (1985).
5. Goldie, N. (1977) 'The Division of Labour among Mental Health Professions – a negotiated or an imposed order?' in Stacey, M. et al. (eds) *Health and the Division of Labour*, Tavistock, London.
6. Miller, P. (1981) 'Psychiatry, the Negotiation of a Territory', a review of Castel, F. et al., *Power and Desire, Diagrams of the Social*, in *Ideology and Consciousness*, no. 8, Spring.
7. *Mental Health Case in the Dutch Welfare State*, 7–10 April 1983, Utrecht.
8. Holland, S. (1979) 'The Development of an Action and Counselling Service in a Deprived Urban Area', *New Methods of Mental Health Care*, Molly Meacher (ed), Pergamon Press.
9. Cockburn, C. (1977) *The Local State*, Pluto Press.
10. Hogget, P., Lousada J. (1985) 'Therapeutic Interventions in Working Class Communities', *Free Associations*, 1, Free Association Books.
11. Banton, R. et al. (1985) *The Politics of Mental Health, Critical Texts in Social Work and the Welfare State*, Macmillan, London.
12. Whittington, C., Holland, R. (1985) 'A Framework for Theory in Social Work', *Issues in Social Work Education*, vol. 5, no. 1 (Summer 1985).
13. Burrell, G., Morgan, G. (1979) *Sociological Paradigms and Organisational Analysis*, Heinemann, London.
14. Freire, P. (1972) *Pedagogy of the Oppressed*, Penguin, Harmondworth.
15. Holland, S., Holland, R. (1985) 'Depressed Women: Outposts of Empire and Castles of Skin', Richards, B., *Capitalism and Infancy*, Free Association Books.
16. Ingleby, D. (1976) 'Sanity, Madness and the Welfare State', in Wadsworth, M.J. and Robinson, D., *Studies in Everyday Medical Life*, Martin Robertson.

17. Khan, M. (1983) *Hidden Selves: Between Theory and Practice in Psychoanalysis*, Hogarth Press, London.
18. Rowe, D. (1985) *Living with the Bomb*, Routledge & Kegan Paul, London.

12

Children with Handicaps in Ordinary Schools

ENRICO SALVI, MARCO CECCHINI

Work towards the integration of children with handicaps, which replaces traditional child psychiatry, has been one of the experiences specific to Arezzo since 1971, when the first law which enabled integration was passed by the Italian parliament.[1] However, it was only with the passing of the second – and more comprehensive law – in 1977, that the rest of Italy followed the pioneering examples of Arezzo and Perugia.[2]

The need to discuss the various stages of marginalization of these children – foundling hospitals, special schools, medical/educational institutes, psychiatric hospitals – arose from the presence of four-year-olds in mental hospitals. There they were diagnosed as 'a danger to oneself, others and an outrage to the public'.

The change took place within the framework of the schools crisis at the end of the 1960s. This period saw the beginnings of mass education and the struggle against selectionism and neglect. It became possible to entertain the choice of integrated classes, with the development of teachers' new professionality; families saw this as the end of experiences where they had been stigmatized and made to feel guilty and ashamed.

In 1971[3] the mental health service in Arezzo (MHS) began to develop both integration of handicapped children in normal classrooms and a new approach to psychological and therapeutic care of handicapped children based on the following main points:

- The shaping of interactions between the parents and their handicapped child inside the family, in order to reduce overprotection and refusal attitudes and to promote more realistic and rewarding attitudes on the parents' side;
- A careful analysis of the child's spontaneous behaviour in different normal settings, in order to understand the causes of fluctuations in

motivation and spontaneous purposeful behaviour;

- A careful analysis of the level of the child's intrinsic motivation in the activities proposed by the therapist, avoiding low motivating activities. Therapeutic work was carried on mainly in the normal settings (home, classroom, playground, holidays);
- Reduction of role fragmentation between the MHS professionals (psychologists, social workers, physio- and speech therapists) to a minimum level;
- A total avoidance of psychotropic and sedative drugs. Difficult behaviours could be handled by understanding their psychological causes.

In Arezzo integration in nursery and primary schools started on a voluntary basis. Parents of handicapped children attending nursery or primary special schools and classrooms were requested by professionals of the MHS if they would have their children leave the special school (or classroom) to be integrated in normal classrooms, mainly according to the children's chronological age.

By 1973 handicapped children who started schooling in normal classrooms in nurseries at the age of three and in primary schools at the age of six, were the first children with no experience of special schooling. They were attending the school nearest to their home in order to:

- Have an increase of interactions with neighbours, peers and families;
- Have no more than one handicapped child per class;
- Reach an even distribution of problems among schools;
- Attain a decrease in transport costs.

Teachers too were chosen on a voluntary basis. Between 1971 and 1975 attendance at state special schools and classrooms – nursery and primary – dropped by 75 per cent and since 1975 new enrolments in special schools and classes ended for lack of request.

Working Practices

The main aim of treatment for young people is to try to overcome difficulties presented by damage, abnormalities or insufficient stimulation. We are also constantly engaged in finding the appropriate level of communication. We want to activate resources in the environment by involving and changing the attitudes of people engaged in the fields of life/study/work. Our experience has taught us that early intervention, a global approach, continuity, a multidisciplinary approach and systematic monitoring of results are necessary prerequisites for success.

Any indication that a child is experiencing real difficulties is related to the team. This team will then examine the needs and requests of the individual in his/her situation in order to establish which worker is most suited to the case. In this way treatment is not fragmented within various professions and/or within the various fields which the child experiences. The team's collective monitoring of results obtained, prevents any worker feeling 'isolated' and guarantees flexible and varied methods of treatment.

To summarize, the relationship between health/social services/ school takes the following course:

- A consultation in order to understand the child, his/her capabilities, difficulties, the strategies s/he adopts, and the dynamics he/she sets in motion or takes part in;
- An agreed programme for creating the necessary conditions for integration of the child with a handicap. This includes the provision of the necessary types of school support, provision of various services (for example, transport, welfare, benefits) when necessary. It also implies action for guaranteeing continuity of method from nursery to primary and to middle school;
- Direct responsibility taken on behalf of the child/family for diagnosis and rehabilitative treatment either on social/health service premises or at home;
- Identification of health education topics to be developed and presented to the whole school population (pupils, teachers, parents) connected with research into epidemiology. This will pinpoint areas of risk or harm and make it possible to define preventive measures.

The debate on achievement (scholastic–social–emotional) has been characterized by the fact that no fixed standard of attainment was specified. Individuals with handicaps were not classified by type but detailed attention was paid to their different starting points. However, at the present time this debate is replaced by focusing individual levels of achievement according to the agreed school programme.

During the schools crisis of the 1970s, the relationship between school–community–society was made the centre of attention. The objectives and functions of separate worlds, each with its own way of self-government, came up against a hypothesis whereby each could be integrated with the other. The focusing of attention on conditions of everyday life required a unified approach to the production of goods, the production of values and consensus and the reproduction of life. The speed of change in the modern world has called into question established knowledge. The result has been recognition of a modern need, i.e. the need to 'learn how to learn' in order to be able to respond to continually changing conditions of life. We must also remember that we live with the restructuring of production based on mass unemployment, delayed entry into the world of work and a lengthening of the period of youth dependency. The response in schools seems to be a return to selective methods and objectives – a response which indicates a function which from a sociocultural point of view has been increasingly discredited. Against this background of social change, school integration became a necessary requirement for individuals with handicaps in their progress towards acquiring autonomy in the 1970s.

It combined with other factors in schools to overcome the:

- Ineffectiveness of the standardization of learning;
- Separation by culture and methodology between nursery, primary and middle school, as well as between class teacher and support teacher;
- Isolation of teachers within the same network or band of parallel classes;
- Competitiveness between pupils in order to encourage solidarity and co-operation.

In this way, integrating handicapped pupils became part of a process to change the framework of 'normalness' . In such a framework where the diversity of one individual enriches the other, deviation becomes a part of the whole, not a proportion to be expelled.

Taking action against selection meant paying attention to the various ways of expressing needs. It meant attempting to adapt and change relationships in the environment in order to confer greater dignity on non-traditional means of expression (for example, body language as well as reading/writing/arithmetic). And all this required a change in the pace, methods and organization of schools. In fact, it is still thought that integrating pupils who are demotivated or with a handicap requires a revision of educational methods and content and a more open, flexible network of school structures which relates to the needs of the majority.

The following themes have been developed in particular over the course of the years:

- How to implement a psychological teaching programme;

- The type of liaison between teachers and social/health services;
- The function of support teachers;
- Common, motivating activities for all children in relation to specific help for individuals experiencing difficulties.

In particular, support teaching needed to be handled with care. Otherwise we ran the risk of re-establishing segregation inside the class in the guise of remedial teaching. In fact, most pupils with a handicap did not wish to be singled out by having a support teacher. By painstaking observation of support teachers' work and of each other's and pupils' reactions, the teachers were helped to learn for themselves how to support the integration of the child best and how to increase his/her motivation to learn. Support teaching is provided usually for six hours per week per child. This amount is increased if the disability is severe.

Some of the encouraging main results of our hypothesis show that:

- On the child's side there is a high motivation towards attending school, meeting the therapist, performing proposed games and tasks, independently from the syndrome and the age at which the integration started. One evident effect of this high degree of motivation is that the move from primary to lower secondary is seen as a rewarding step to be achieved. Quite often these pupils have been more confident in their ability to cope with the new situations than the therapists themselves.
- On the peers' side there have been very few episodes of overt rejection of the handicapped child by his peers inside the normal classrooms, and these have been mainly due to behavioural problems. Understanding the child's problems and modification of the negative attitudes on the teachers' or on the parents' side (either peers' or the child's parents) was enough to modify the situation. Episodes of active solidarity between peers and the handicapped children have been very frequent. There are no demonstrated negative effects on the school performance of pupils who had a handicapped child in their classroom for up to five years.
- On the teachers' side the changes in attitude have been quite complex. In Arezzo today there is no overt criticism of integration either from groups of teachers or from their unions. Some retired teachers offered their voluntary help in upper secondary schools, where peripatetic teachers don't exist. Spontaneous peer relationships have led also to:

- The discovery of ways of communicating with autistic children;
- Suggestions for cognitive and instrumental activities which emerged outside normal lessons;
- Using free time and/or doing homework at the homes of handicapped pupils or their friends' homes.

The difficulties of teachers regarding changes in their role have been the subject of continual attention by the school and the administrative sectors. Many meetings aimed at preventing such difficulties becoming 'personal' problems, and thereby directly affecting the relationship with handicapped pupils, took place. With this aim in mind, institutional programming has taken on a fundamental role. This programme is responsible for monitoring activities undertaken jointly by school management/services and the families aimed at preparing the class and teaching staff before the start of the new school year.

Increasingly, teachers are liaising from nursery to primary to middle school. This is achieved by visiting the individual sections/classes in which these pupils are placed in order to ensure the continuity of methods and teaching styles. School meetings take place with the parents of these children, apart from the meetings of the different workers involved. These parents can also attend the regular meeting for parents of all children in the class or meet with their elected delegates or representative bodies.

The current national situation is illustrated in information collated by the national enquiry undertaken by the Studies and Programme Office from the Ministry of Public Education on the subject of nursery schools and state obligations in the year 1979–80. The data shows that:

- The number of children in special education reached its peak around 1970 and has been declining since. In 1980 the number of children in special schools in all of Italy was 14,838, compared with 71,751 in 1970. Special classes did not exist in 1980, whereas in 1970 there were 63,565 children in such classes. In the Arezzo area – with 320,000 inhabitants – there were 97 children in special education in 1980, compared with 483 in 1970.[4]
- Integration of children with handicaps in ordinary school is much more marked in the north and centre than in the south of Italy. Thus 44 per cent of all pupils in the north's ordinary classes are allocated to children with handicaps, 38 per cent in the centre and 20.2 per cent in the south. The south leads the list of continuous availability of special education.[5]

Integrating the handicapped, as well as promoting 'rehabilitation' for the handicapped individual, is also beneficial to health care for all children. This is because it increases the opportunities for debate, information and education concerning health by using specific situations and themes.

By paying attention to local and national administration of family planning and prenatal care which will pinpoint high risk cases at the earliest opportunity, handicaps can be reduced. A preventive health care service needs functional links between all structures which are concerned at national and local level with child care and the interconnections between illness, damage, disability, limitation, handicap and context.

This approach to a whole array of factors occurring in everyday life enables the real implementation of primary, secondary and tertiary prevention concerning children. Preventive care not only increases 'tolerance' of diversity amongst pupils, teachers and parents but diversity becomes positively understood and accepted.

However, when compulsory schooling for the first integrated pupils was completed, the very serious lack of employment and recreational opportunities and the problems of youth disadvantage were brought into focus. Lack of action in these sectors means that any effort towards achieving independence and self-sufficiency risks failure and dissipation. And that all the various forms through which 'the condition of the young' expresses itself are in danger of being prolonged and increased. A whole range of problems are being increasingly highlighted – from extra-curricular activities to the use of free time, from how the young live within the community to which venues can be used throughout the year, for meetings, cultural and recreational activities.

The reality is that plans for non-segregational and non-discriminatory acceptance into employment have proceeded no further than being accepted in principle by young people, families, workers, unions and employee organizations in the working world. The statutory provision for employment of the handicapped is calmly evaded and positive experiences are sporadic.

Concerted joint action on behalf of handicapped individuals – in order to avoid entering institutions and chronic dependence on health and social services – has been made difficult by the scarcity of resources and by the restructuring process currently being experienced by those in employment.

One response to the difficulties encountered by those attempting to make provision for needs traditionally neglected (i.e. the restriction of space, opportunities and direct expression of need as alternatives to those needs simply being interpreted) has been the emergence of family associations. These associations are pressure groups aiming at ensuring provision of adequate resources from appropriate political bodies. However, these attempts to change the quality of everyday community life are increasingly being presented as idealistic and are countered by requests for new types of custody and containment.

What we are trying to continue doing is to leave behind the blind alleys of impotence and the thinking which postpones action. Instead we are creating collective responsibility and solidarity in specific environments; we are trying to link professional practice to accepted social practice in freeing resources and overcoming obstacles in the path of handicap and misery and deprivation. All this must take place as a response to needs and the debate must be opened up about the increasingly widespread separation of the political process.

All too often, between cuts in social spending and crises in the welfare state

the only concern is to give a technical response, as a means of implementing the normalization process: life within the family, school integration, accommodation, work, free time. These responses must not be ends in themselves but are a phase in the struggle for a change in everyday life.[6]

References

1. The 1971 law is Law no. 118/71. On the experience of Arezzo see: De Leonardis, O. (1982) *Dopo il Manicomio*, Il Pensiero Scientifico, Rome. Ramon, S. (1983) '*Psichiatria Democratica*: A Case Study of an Italian Community Mental Health Service', *International Journal of Health Services*, 13, 2, pp. 307–24. Martini, P. et al. (1985) 'A model of a single comprehensive Mental Health Service for a catchment area: a community alternative to hospitalisation', *Acta Psychiatrica Scandinavica*, vol. 71, supplement, pp. 96–120.

2. Law 1977 is Law no. 517/77. While Law 118/71 focuses on the definition of handicap, Law 517/77 focuses on the educational issues of integration and the regulations required to achieve it. For the impact in other parts of Italy see: Vislie, L. (1980) *Integration of Handicapped Children in Italy: A View from the Outside*, OECD, Paris.

3. See Bruzzone, A.M. (1979) *Ci Chiamarano Matti*, Einaudi, Milan.

4. Italian Bureau of Statistics, 1981.

5. Ibid.

6. Quoted from the conclusions of the working party on 'Social policy for minors and the experiences of working with people with handicaps' at the International Network for Alternatives to Psychiatry congress, Rome, May 1985.

13
British Special Hospitals

DAVID PILGRIM

Much has been written about the British special hospitals. This has tended to fall into two categories. The first has been written by clinicians working within the system who have produced either uncritical or defensive descriptions.[1] In the second category are critical thoughts provided by observers. Although these have appeared from both civil libertarian positions[2] and official reports (see later), they are dismissed by those involved with the preservation of the special hospitals as unreliable or uninformed. An understandably defensive stance of those depending for their livelihoods on an isolated system under frequent attack is to claim that those outside fail to appreciate the nature of problems suffered by those working on the inside. This defence may not be particularly valid but it is intelligible and therefore has to be acknowledged as part of the problem of having a free and open debate about a system which is manifestly a victim of its own history.

These problems of free debate will be picked up again below along with various other difficulties that have accumulated inside the special hospitals over time. Before this critical overview is presented, however, some attempt will be made to give an outline of the main features of the system.

An Outline of the Special Hospital System

There are four special hospitals in England, which are administered directly by the Department of Health and Social Security (DHSS). Except for Park Lane, which was opened in 1984, the established institutions were built piecemeal during this century or wholly in Victorian times like Broadmoor. In addition Carstairs State Hospital serves a similar function but is administered by the Scottish Home and Health Board. Two of the English hospitals, Moss Side and Park Lane, share a campus 8 miles north of Liverpool. Rampton Hospital is in the Nottinghamshire countryside, 15 miles to the west of Lincoln.

Broadmoor is in a greenbelt of Berkshire, 10 miles from Reading.

All of these hospitals contain residents (called 'patients' by most staff) who at some time in their history relevant to admission decisions have been adjudged to be suffering from violent, dangerous or criminal propensities in addition to being mentally disordered. Under present legislation the legal/clinical labels for these residents always involves one or more of the following: mental illness; psychopathic disorder; mental impairment; severe mental impairment. The hospitals have developed a specialist interest to some degree. Broadmoor and Park Lane tend not to admit mentally handicapped patients. The numbers in this category will reduce given that the changes in the Mental Health Act (1983) now make it necessary for patients to manifest proven dangerousness in addition to handicap which used not to be the case. This and other tightening of admission criteria have meant that over the past 20 years, the system has been operating at a net loss of patients. Over the past ten years patient numbers have more than halved. The All Party Social Services Committee spells out the cost implications of this as follows:

> The DHSS will be spending around £50 million in 1985–6 on the four Special Hospitals ... In 1981–2, the hospitals cost around £31 million net; in 1982–3, around £35 million; in 1983–4 around £42 million; and in 1984–5 around £45 million. The Special Hospitals contain around 1,600 patients. It costs at present around £30,000 a year to care for a Special Hospital patient, or almost £600 per week. (para 6, page viii, 1985 report)

Thus a very expensive system is numerically running down but is escalating in costs. The reduction in admission rates and total residents may lead to two misunderstandings. The hospitals contain a core of patients (certain murderers, paedophiles and rapists) who by common agreement will remain incarcerated for many years. This core, the size of which is debated, pre-empts the system reaching a predictable point of closedown. (Contrary to common opinion, most patients do not fall into this intractable category.) The second misapprehension that may arise is that special hospitals are easy places to leave. This is not the case. Most residents stay for periods of time commensurate with the severity of their index offence.[3] This does not reflect an explicit policy (most patients are admitted under sections of the Mental Health Act which may entail detention without specified limit). What this does reflect is the penal ideology that governs decision making within the system.

Moreover, even when transfer or discharge has been agreed, many patients fail to move on because of poor aftercare facilities. The latter may be a function of inadequate resources or of facilities being present but whose managers refuse to take these patients. Consequently, these aftercare problems have led to around 16 per cent of special hospital patients being held inside even though their transfer or discharge has been agreed.[4]

Inside the hospitals, basic daily activities are similar to any other long-stay institution. In addition to custody and the daily round of medication rituals, patients have access to various educational and occupational activities. The latter do not appear to facilitate post-discharge employment, however.[5] Moreover, psychologically orientated therapies are sparse and for reasons to be outlined below are subject to sabotage.

One imbalance within the special hospital population relates to the impact of past and present admission policies. As was mentioned above, admission criteria have become tighter over the years. Now the DHSS are keen that only those proven to be a grave and immediate danger to others will be admitted. However, such stringency was not applied in the past, so that many who have become trapped in the system would now be refused admission if their original deviance was being evaluated. (Attention is drawn to the notion of original deviance as a recognition that deviance may amplify inside closed institutions – this plus the disabling impact of being cut off from everyday experiences in the community are the two main components of 'institutionalization'.) Another imbalance within the population relates to the type of resident contained. Most psychiatric services contain more women than men. The reverse is true inside special hospitals, with a ratio of four to one 'favouring' male residents. This probably reflects the wider issue of these hospitals containing population seen as likely to be residents. It should be noted however that not all patients are offenders (at Broadmoor around a fifth of the residents are non-offenders).[6] Also the special hospitals not only take court referrals and prison transfers but in addition they act as a 'back-stop' for NHS hospitals that have problems managing disturbed patients.

As far as the organization of the special hospital system is concerned there are certain peculiarities that need highlighting. The hospitals have a local management on site and are visited twice yearly by a management committee from the DHSS in London. This centralized and distant management has been criticized repeatedly over the years and culminated in a second tier of local management being instituted at Rampton and more recently (1986) small health boards at Moss Side, Park Lane and Broadmoor have been suggested but not implemented. Two government departments other than the DHSS are involved in the system. The Department of the Environment is responsible for maintaining the physical structures of the hospitals and the Home Office is regularly involved in making decisions about offender-patients in terms of their discharge or transfer.

The employees of the hospitals including the clinical staff have civil service status which means that they are subjected to the constraints of the Official Secrets Act and specific regulations concerning the publication of material, a key determinant probably in the character of publications pointed out in the first paragraph. (These constraints to a degree are influencing what is being said and not being said in this chapter – note the disclaimer at the end.)

Another way that the special hospitals are peculiar is that the nursing and occupations staff, except at the new hospital of Park Lane, wear prison officer type uniforms. A one-off visit to these hospitals gives the impression that they are little distinguishable from prisons; a view that can be argued by more informed critics. Until recently only the Prison Officers' Association was recognized for collective bargaining purposes as a trade union. Staff organizations within the NHS have not been accepted by the DHSS as far as the special system is concerned, though at the time of writing, the ASTMS trade union has been recognized to represent clinical psychologists following many years of lobbying and failed attempts to gain recognition.

Now that a description has been given of the special hospitals an attempt will be made to draw together a set of criticisms most of which are elaborated elsewhere.[7]

Criticisms

Though they are formally managed as healthcare institutions, special hospitals are most accurately understood as prisons for the mad, the incorrigibly bad and the unintelligibly dim. They are different from typical prisons in two main senses. First, a prisoner is usually given a specified sentence whereas a special hospital patient is not. The patient's ongoing behaviour during their hospital career is often matched against their index offence, and ordinary institutional behaviour (homosexuality or fighting) is frequently attributed to individual characteristics of the patient. In a prison infractions of institutional rules at most lead to loss of remission. In the context of a hospital such rule breaking is often framed as pathology.

Patients rarely enjoy the social validation that the solidarity of the 'inmate code' brings to prisoners. To offset these mystifications, and the isolation of special hospital patient status, the standards of welfare and rehabilitation in British prisons (with laudable exceptions like Grendon Underwood) are very poor. Consequently, many individuals who are vulnerable to psychological distress enjoy a more benign material environment in a special hospital than in a typical prison. The discrepancy in such standards should not be exaggerated however. Until Park Lane was built to absorb the overcrowding at Broadmoor the latter provided prison levels of material deprivation:

The European Commission of Human Rights held admissible a complaint that the conditions and treatment provided in Broadmoor Hospital constituted a violation of article 3 of the European Convention in that they were inhuman and degrading (Smith vs. the UK, 1981).[8]

Two years prior to this ruling the special hospital system was subjected to its most damning public condemnation to date. In May 1979, Yorkshire Television screened a programme entitled *The Secret Hospital*, in which allegations of widespread brutality on the part of nursing staff against patients were reported. Over 100 nurses were reported to be involved in the assaults. Nearly 1,000 cases were presented to the Director of Public Prosecutions. The programme was about Rampton Hospital which was immediately subjected to a managerial review under the chairmanship of Sir John Boynton. The Boynton Report[9] was 175 pages long and contained 205 recommendations for change at Rampton.

This picture is bad enough but the main factor that condemns the system relates to the impact (or lack of it) of previous reports. Previously, in 1971, the Hospital Advisory Service had drawn attention to problems that Boynton found unresolved. Likewise, the Elliott Report sponsored but not published by the DHSS found similar problems in 1973.[10] As Morris[11] pertinently asks 'why were Elliott's fears ignored?' This picture of inaction on the part of central management was not peculiar to Rampton. As Martin[12] has highlighted when tracing patterns of organization in degrading institutions, often state departments and even ministers know that severe problems exist inside institutions ostensibly designed to provide care, yet they fail to act. Such is the inertia of large organizations and the bureaucracies that govern them that knowledge may fail to avert brutality.

It is an inadequate rationalization on the part of the defenders of the existing system to reduce the problems at Rampton to the issue of the existence of a few sadistic staff. Martin demonstrates that such a component is swamped by recurrent organizational features within hospitals that have contained neglect and brutality. For this reason a second rationalization also fails – that the special hospitals hold the most difficult patients in the country. This cannot explain brutality in itself as other hospitals have manifested similar problems (though maybe not to the same degree) where only frail or handicapped patients are held.

A common feature of these hospitals is that they contain long-term populations and they are organizationally isolated. Thus if any factor can be seen to predominate it is the segregation of deviant populations and of the staff for long periods of time. More specifically, the special hospitals are counter-therapeutic in the following ways:

- They are organizationally and professionally isolated;
- They subordinate therapy to security (Martin describes this as the 'corruption of care');[13]
- A prison trade union operates a constant negative veto on clinical matters;
- Because of their national catchment, patients are often dislocated from their social network and area of origin (though at times this protects them from vengeful neighbourhoods);
- They contain a poor stock of knowledge of softer forms of intervention like psychotherapy. Instead custody and chemotherapy predominate (it is debatable though whether this picture differs significantly from other large psychiatric hospitals);
- The maximum security ethos means that there is worst contingency planning, i.e. most patients are subjected to the same level of security and the restrictions that brings;
- The size of the hospitals involves a rotating shift system that disrupts continuity of care at ward level;
- As large organizational units they are associated with poor internal communication and paranoid processes;[14]
- They are isolated from corrective feedback from without.

On this last point, it is true that some ongoing feedback is now being provided by the Mental Health Act Commission (MHAC). This was set up following the 1983 Mental Health Act. What is unclear is the degree to which the Commission will get drawn in and entangled with the system. If this does happen and corrective influence fails to occur, then the MHAC will have become part of the problem rather than part of the solution. It is early days to evaluate the impact of the MHAC. One issue is certain. The Commission cannot reverse the problems inherent to large organizational units and geographical isolation. Such problems can only be solved by abolishing the present system.

In the light of the counter-therapeutic features outlined above, MIND have campaigned to phase out the special hospitals and have them replaced by smaller locally managed units offering flexible security tailored to patient needs. Governments of both political hues have failed to respond to such an abolitionist lobby to date. Any perceived liberalization of the existing arrangement for mentally abnormal offenders is likely to win few votes. The most optimistic scenario that MIND is likely to achieve is the eventual abolition of the three older hospitals. Park Lane is likely to remain open for two reasons. It has recently cost over £30 million to build and it is the appropriate size for the core group of intractable residents mentioned earlier. The pessimistic scenario of little or no change in the forseeable future is implied by the willingness of the state to invest more in the older hospitals. (Presently Rampton and Broadmoor are being rebuilt.) Only a clearcut political decision to accept the MIND lobby will override these recent investments.

The MIND blueprint is essentially an extension of the Regional Secure Unit system recommended by the Butler Report in 1975.[15] However, even this reform has remained largely on paper, with local health authorities failing to finance new units even when central funding was allocated and nurses refusing to work in them. By 1983, only 20 beds were open out of 717 planned places.[16]

A crucial question is begged by this picture of variable financing of projects related to secure provision. Why is it that at a time when the present government is running down old psychiatric hospitals to save money the special hospitals are being given the privilege of investment? Clearly there is something special about the special hospitals – they are a centrally managed form of hard social control. The state is unlikely to renounce such central authority readily. One measure of political commitment to a project is to finance it. This is exactly what our present government is doing generally in the area of hard social control.

At the moment, the DHSS spends £600 per patient per week on the special hospitals (see above). Such is the measure of a commitment to control those who are doubly deviant by dint of being dangerous and mentally disordered. The existence of the specials as hospitals rather than prisons allows politicians to readily gloss over the social control issue. They can frame the expense in terms of a benevolent commitment to the welfare of one group of sick people. As was indicated above, any close scrutiny of the system reveals that it is counter-therapeutic. But provided enough clinical trappings are bought (the hiring of clinical staff, the pills and the white coats over the prison officer type uniforms) politicians are thereby supplied with a basis for rhetoric. This rhetoric assures the public that dangerous people are segregated but in a humane and therapeutic manner.

In Britain, the medicalization of criminality has held out the hope of such a therapeutic outcome. But behind the rhetoric of politicians and staff loyal to the existing system lies a picture of failed hope. The mentally handicapped should not be kept in prison-like conditions. The NHS should be providing local facilities for difficult to manage handicapped patients. If the mad are to lose their liberty, they should do so inside their local psychiatric facilities and discharge decisions should be made on the basis of their psychological state not their index offence.

Those labelled psychopathic, if they do not want any treatment, should be given a custodial prison disposal with a finite sentence. Those requiring access to change should spend such a sentence in a prison offering a psychosocial treatment programme (such as the therapeutic community regime at Grendon). The term 'psychopath' seems to epitomize the worst aspects of the medical model: it has maximal stigma value and minimal therapeutic outcome when medical approaches are used.

Those admitting the failure of standard medical prescriptions for psychopathy sometimes rationalize the present special hospital regime as offering 'milieu therapy'. This is a rather circular way of justifying the authoritarianism of a social system on the grounds that it will have an automatic resocializing influence. All of the literature on institutionalization indicates such a system typically damages rather than rehabilitates. Autonomy and self-responsibility are not fostered by authoritarian regimes: conformity to the institutional rules and dependency may be fostered however.

Finally some comment needs to be made on the civil liberties of staff inside the special hospital system. The civil servant status of clinicians at first sight poses few problems but problems there are. The graduate professions in particular are socialized to expect a degree of academic freedom of expression. Such expression from within the special hospitals is obstructed by three features. First there are anxieties generated by being subject to the Official Secrets Act.

A similar set of anxieties are produced by civil service regulations on publication. These are the legacy of a tradition that encourages loyalty to and diplomacy about the state structures that give civil servants their employment. Loyalty and diplomacy are admirable qualities in their appropriate context. In other contexts they are the ready basis for duplicity, hypocrisy and rhetoric; in short mystification. A system that is advertised as therapeutic but that fails in its promise demands a frank exposure. The very existence of an apparatus to impede such an exposure implies that there is or there might be something to hide.

The third impediment to an open debate about the special hospitals involves the threat or the occurrence of industrial action on the part of the Prison Officers' Association. This occurred at Moss Side in early 1985 when the Prison Officers' Association instructed its members to withdraw co-operation with my clinical work, for publishing an article critical of the present system.[17] Similarly, at Rampton following the Boynton Report the Prison Officers' Association imposed reporting restrictions confirming the very accusation of closed defensiveness that critics of the hospital had recurrently made. These three impediments to free speech discourage unhappy clinicians from speaking out. None of this is very surprising. People cannot expect soft treatment from institutions of hard social control.

Author's note: The views in this chapter are personal and do not represent the official opinion of Moss Side Hospital or the DHSS.

References

1. Hamilton, J. (1986) 'The Special Hospitals', in Gostin, L. (ed) *Secure Provision*, Tavistock, London, 1985; Hendry, M. (1983) 'Nursing Behind Bars', *Nursing Mirror*, 2 March, pp. 16–18
2. Gostin, L. (ed) (1985) *Secure Provision*.
3. Norris, M. (1984) *Integration of Special Hospital Patients into the Community*, Gower, London.
4. Gostin, L. (ed) (1985) *Secure Provision*.
5. Norris, M. (1984) *Integration of Special Hospital Patients into the Community*.
6. Ibid.
7. Pilgrim D., Eisenberg N. (1985) 'Should Special Hospitals be phased out?' *Bulletin of the British Psychological Society*, 38, pp. 281–4; Pilgrim, D. (1984) 'Whither the Special Hospitals?' *Open Mind*, 12, 14 December.
8. Gostin, L. (1983) 'The Ideology of Entitlement' in P. Bean, *Mental Illness: Changes and Trends* Wiley, Chichester.
9. Boynton, J. (1980) *Report of the Review of Rampton Hospital*, DHSS, HMSO, London.
10. Elliott, J. (1973) *Report on Rampton Hospital* (DHSS unpublished).
11. Morris, P. (1979) 'Why were Elliott's fears ignored?' *Nursing Mirror*, 7 June, 6.

12. Martin, J.P. (1984) *Hospitals in Trouble*, Blackwell, Oxford.

13. Ibid.

14. deBoard, R. (1978) *The Psychoanalysis of Organisations*, Tavistock, London.

15. Butler, R.A. (1975) *Report of the Committee on Mentally Abnormal Offenders*, DHSS, HMSO, London.

16. Snowden, P.R. (1983) 'The Regional Secure Unit Programme: a Personal Appraisal', *Bulletin of the Royal College of Psychiatrists*, 7 August (8), pp. 138–40.

17. Pilgrim, D. (1984) 'Whither the Special Hospitals?' *Open Mind*, 12, 14 December.

14

The Judicial Psychiatric Hospital: a Difficult Reform?

GIOVANNA DEL GIUDICE, PASQUALE EVARISTO, MARIA GRAZIA GIANNICHEDDA

The Juridical Form and the Institutional Function of the Judicial Psychiatric Hospital

Judicial Psychiatric Hospitals (JPHs) developed from the first separate section for the insane in prison, which appeared in 1876, in Aversa (southern Italy). In 1891, the penal code rationalized the JPH as a place of internment for 'those who became mentally ill in prison and those diagnosed as suffering from mental infirmity'. This separation was seen as an attempt to free the prison from madness. Jurists and psychiatrists shared the pressure for the separation, aimed by the latter at eliminating the dangerous patients from the psychiatric hospital. This process of selection and expulsion from the two institutions resulted in the emergence of the JPH. Therefore its function is clearly related to the internal logic and conceptual trends of the penal and psychiatric systems: it becomes their point of balance.

With the penal code of 1931, admission to the JPH assumes an actual juridical form: the mentally infirm person is 'condemned' to be 'cured' in the JPH for a minimum of two, five or ten years, depending on the offence s/he is accused of and for which s/he was not tried due to illness. The intricate ambiguity of therapy and juridical sanctions is thus legitimized. The punishment becomes simultaneously excluding and threatening, the therapy postulated and negated. The JPH is placed under the responsibility of the Ministry of Justice, i.e. the personnel consists mainly of prison officers, and even the medical staff depends on the prison administration. The physical structure of the JPH resembles a prison. The goal of cure not only does not sweeten the regime but perhaps makes it worse, by enabling a further suspension of personal rights. Until the beginning of the 1970s the JPH was in fact used as a threat against the most undisciplined prisoners: about half of the total prison population was condemned to 'psychiatric observation' for fixed periods.

When some magistrates exposed the case of the JPH in the 1960s, the function of this institution was questioned. On the one hand it is a 'forgotten' remnant of the Fascist regime and a unique case among the present European laws. On the other hand it had an original function and still has one, if it is true that all of the Western laws maintain special institutions aimed at containing the 'incongruent subjects' expelled from prison and the psychiatric hospital.

The negative judgement of this penal code (known as Rocco's Code) is still shared today. But no reform of it took place, apart from a few decisions by the Constitutional Court, the role of which is to judge in cases of conflict between the principles of the Italian constitution and the way it is practised in other courts. There are two reasons for this:

- The penal reform approved in 1975 did not touch the JPH because a psychiatric reform was expected. When, three years later, the psychiatric reform was legislated for, the laws concerning terrorism had created a sociopolitical atmosphere which favoured closure of the penal institution and its administrative elements.
- The debate during the 1970s and the analysis of foreign experiences have led to doubts: if the assumption of the need for a special institution for the mentally ill offender is maintained, is it possible to avoid the production of a total institution which negates in reality what it affirms in principle? How are we to ensure that this prison/hospital does not end up being a no man's land, a zone free of rights and of medicine, a place which constructs for the inmates the destiny of inability to be cured under the banner of the most human response? Finally, how can we avoid that the aberration of the penal code, cancelled at the level of civil rights, will not be reproduced at the level of institutional management?

In reality, while no decisions have been made on these issues, the aim of abolishing the JPH has begun to be expressed and is currently the most frequently-debated possibility. This option is also the most difficult in relation to the real configuration of the two systems.

The present Italian debate is extremely interesting from this angle. The only group which continues to be interested in the problem of the JPH are those who think that it is both necessary and possible to abolish it. They are the judges, psychiatrists and researchers of the two subject areas. They have developed further the concepts of imputability and ability to reason and at the practical level are using the openings made available by the Constitutional Court's decisions (see below). Those who think that it is necessary to retain the JPH or its equivalents tend to use as an excuse the deplorable state of the Italian prisons and the weakness of community psychiatry, avoiding discussion of any 'uncomfortable' cases. To summarize, in the country of Lombroso and Ferri, where the illusion of an anthropology of crime as a medical science prevailed, the principal justification of a special institution for 'mentally ill offenders' is the conviction that in reality it is impossible to move the prison and the psychiatric systems towards the rights and needs of people. This 'realism' is then used to justify accepting the distance between laws and institutions, even when it is the weakest who pay the price.

Hospitalization in the JPH: Penal and Health Legislation

The penal law currently regulating hospitalization in the JPH is still the 1931 Act. The sharp contrast between that law, the constitution and Law 180 led the Constitutional Court to pass several sentences which have modified certain aspects of the penal code and that which regulates the procedure. Thus a paradox exists: the aberrations of the penal code are still valid, but the Court's decision enables psychiatry to reduce drastically entry to the JPH and to discharge those still there. As the case description below demonstrates, this is already happening in those situations where the psychiatric model presented in this book is practised.

This fact provides a final confirmation of the hypothesis that these people (the 'mad' criminal, for example) have no special characteristics which justify the existence of a special institution. Above all, it proves that with the ideological and practical change in the two systems, it is possible to exclude this group without serious damage to the social order or the well-being of the individual.

In order to understand the terms of the problem a delineation of the major modifications offered by the Constitutional Court is required: since the war, the six Italian JPHs have had a population of 1,500 to 1,800 a year. About half of these are defined as 'mentally infirm', because of their psychiatric condition. They are those who, although found guilty of an offence, are said to be 'unable to have acted intentionally and willingly'. The need for secure provision, namely internment in the JPH, arises out of this inability.

Until 1982 the decision of total infirmity led automatically to the application of psychiatric secure provision. Unable equalled dangerous: it was an absolute declaration of dangerousness about anyone who was declared infirm as a result of illness.

The court, responding to 21 exceptions presented by different lower courts after Law 180 was approved, has decided that following Law 180, 'dangerousness' when an offence was committed is no longer a sufficient reason for secure provision. Dangerousness needs to be proven at the moment of passing judgment on the offence. Thus a person deemed as unable to act intentionally at the time of the offence may remain 'unable' at the time of the psychiatric investigation for the court, but not necessarily be also dangerous. In the latter case no secure provision is required.

Consequently, when an accused person is found unable to act intentionally, admission to a JPH is no longer a must; s/he can be looked after at his/her place of residence by the local psychiatric service. The same applies in the case of diminished responsibility. While in the case of full inability a judge has the overall responsibility, in the second instance this is no longer required. In terms of sentencing it means that s/he may receive a suspended sentence, domiciliary arrest, or parole under specific conditions. At the theoretical level the court's judgment has a very important effect, with which it is possible to modify the psychiatric culture in terms of the relationships between mental illness and social dangerousness, between behaviour and ability to reason. The psychiatric investigation needs to respond to these objectives, as it becomes insufficient merely to demonstrate the existence of a psychiatric symptom as an indication of dangerousness, without specific indicators demonstrated in the behaviour of the person at the moment of the psychiatric investigation.

It is too soon for a full evaluation of the impact of this decision. However, the following observations can be made.

On several occasions judges have complained of the psychiatrists' tendency to treat the issue of dangerousness only in a formal way, continuing to deduce it from the existence of the psychiatric syndrome. However, at the same time new research shows that it is possible to disassociate incapacity from dangerousness, even in serious syndromes. In practice we see the work of psychiatrists, usually from the public sector but also a few from the university forensic departments, who have indirectly decided to allow even those who have committed serious offences to stay outside the JPH, under the responsibility of the psychiatric services. At the same time, we also see a tendency not to use the presence of a serious psychiatric syndrome to make the person stand trial.

Up to now there has been a considerable reduction in the number of people, seen as infirm, with a serious offence against another person, being put under the supervision of the psychiatric services. This is a positive development, explained by the fact that the professionals involved in this work are those who wish to limit the risk of invalidation and de-responsibility of the person, even when s/he suffers from mental distress. They take into consideration not only the social fear which may be produced in such cases, but above all the psychological harm done to a person who will end up hospitalized and thus absolved of responsibility. These psychiatrists make a relatively greater use of the judgment of capacity to make rational decisions and semi-infirmity. The practical consequences of these choices, which are the juridical process and eventually the judgment, are in fact considered to be less harmful for the person's health than is his/her total de-responsibility. In those cases when detention cannot be avoided, the local mental health service may enter the prison and be responsible for the detained person's health.

The following description provides an illustration of what the new approach can mean in the practice of the psychiatric services.

November 1982: the MHC receives a request from the prison social service in Trieste for transferring A. who is in a JPH to the mental hospital in Trieste. The service has never met A. but the memory and ghost of the crime which he committed in January 1974 emerges straight away: he killed his lover by whom he had had three children. His wife is known by several older workers in the centre as an ex-patient, but the centre has had no contact with her for some time. She lives only on an invalidity pension and has greatly deteriorated.

After several days, the centre contacts the judge supervising the JPH: we reply that the mental hospital no longer exists and that at the present time we are not able to work out an alternative programme for A., but that we will come to meet him. The judge expresses the desire to release A. We also learn that in 1977 A. had seriously injured another inmate who subsequently died because of the wounds he received.

We try to find A.'s wife: she spends her day either in the street or at her daughter's home. She can only say a few words. She is very neglected in her appearance although she likes adorning herself with plastic 'jewellery'.

We look for her daughter: we only succeed in speaking to her husband. He does not know A. but has been his legal guardian since 1978, sending him money regularly from his pension. Our relationship with the guardian is not easy. He is obviously a disturbed person. He does not supply us with clear information and seems to contradict himself. He has a lawyer who takes care of the guardianship.

We try to find the lawyer: he supplies us with copies of the psychiatric assessment made on A. but seems unable to give us more information on the pensions to which A. is entitled (a war pension and an occupational pension). We examine the existing assessment: this provides an incomplete picture of the psychiatric and the personal aspects. He is presented as a 'monster', 'without affection or emotion', within a life history which is never separated from a diagnosis as an incurable, irredeemably dangerous schizophrenic.

On 8 December two workers from the centre, a doctor and a nurse, meet with the supervising judge of the JPH, who supplies a disastrous picture of living conditions inside. We express concern on behalf of the Trieste district psychiatric services about any possible reintroduction to Trieste of A., given his history and the current situation of his family.

In the afternoon we make our way to the JPH. We encounter many problems in obtaining permission to visit: the 'detainee' is not identified straight away because his Slavic name has been Italianized and distorted. The motive for the visit is questioned. We get the feeling that we are regarded as being powerless and are identified with the person who we want to visit.

We see A. in the presence of a nurse. Our immediate impression is that he has an extreme need for human contact. He talks about himself a great deal and does not ask us many questions. All he needs to know is that we come from Trieste. He realizes that we may be able to take an interest in him and he asks us to free him from the 'hell' he lives in. He cannot understand why he is still there since he has already served his sentence. He shows precise knowledge of the laws and seems to know and be interested in current issues. He condemns the 'Basaglia Reform' for having forgotten the psychiatric prisons. He keeps recounting his experience of persecution past and present in the psychiatric prison.

He expresses emotion in a few instances only, when the tension drops: asks after his mother; tells us his story of being caught between a jealous and possessive lover and a wife who was no longer able to look after herself. We promise him we will come back to visit him.

We look for his mother: she is more than 80 years old. She is the only person who has continued to maintain a stable relationship with him by sending him money.

17–18 March: we return to the JPH and talk with the magistrate and the deputy director, who is only interested in showing us the new medical clinics which he is creating at the JPH.

We have a conversation with A. and the next day we get permission to take him into town. Outside, he does not need to talk so much about being persecuted but refers to the many violent episodes which marked his life inside mental hospitals.

He speaks of the 'wall of delirium' which he built 'brick by brick' out of the days of imprisonment which were all identical to one another, and almost excuses himself for it. Many questions are asked about life outside. He talks at length to a worker from the same area as himself; about past personalities, streets, cafés.

In April, a card from A. arrives at the centre. New meetings with his son-in-law and daughter demonstrate the disintegration of their family.

We meet the guardian's lawyer in order to obtain a sum of money for A. for a permit to Trieste which we have included in our programme for him (in fact, the guardian only rarely sends him a little money).

Then we ask the tutelary judge for Trieste to clarify A.'s economic situation and how it is managed by his guardian, and we ask to become involved in restoring the electricity supply to A.'s house which had been cut off because the bill had not been paid.

26 May–2 June: A.'s permit to Trieste is received and he is brought back, initially living on the service's premises. He meets his wife: she does not recognize him at first, then asks him to stay at home with her. In the following days she spends most of the time at the centre with her husband. Then A. meets his daughter and his mother. He makes outings into the town in order to get to know it again and to do some shopping. He asks to see again the place where he killed his lover.

Therapy with a retardant drug is suggested. A. is very reluctant but accepts it only because of the relationship which has been built up in this period. (Then we were to learn that the doctors in the JPH convinced him that the drug was useless, even harmful.) He is accompanied back there for the continuation of his permit by the supervising judge.

Then a meeting with the daughter and the wife takes place (at this point the son-in-law has disappeared from the scene) to discuss A.'s future life in Trieste. The daughter expresses a desire to do something for her father which until now she has found impossible. It is decided that he can live during the permit period at his home with his wife. The service then takes over the responsibility of the relationship with both of them, psychological and medical support, help with putting the house in order again, use of the centre's canteen, possibility of using the centre as a day hospital, relationship with the judge, relationship with the guardian.

End of July, A. finally comes back to Trieste. From then onwards his relationship with the centre was and still is on a daily basis; the aim is to strengthen a relationship of mutual trust and knowledge. The guardian was replaced, once it had been made clear to the judge that the former guardian was seriously inadequate. In this way any potentially dangerous problems concerning A.'s relationship with his son-in-law and daughter were avoided.

A. becomes a person again but expresses quite clearly his disappointment at being undermined by the need for a guardian. He shows he is able to manage his own affairs well, but accepts realistically what the law requires.

Contact with the new guardian who testifies to A.'s economic needs is maintained. In addition, medical support is available; home is cleared and cleaned; support is provided for paying the rent arrears; contact is made with the supervisory magistrate near the JPH for the extension of the permits to stay in Trieste; relationship with the police is established to inform them of the situation.

This man's integration into the centre was possible because he was able to cope with a community to whom he owed his freedom; the professionals were able to cope with him throughout and beyond his life history and illness; the centre was able to provide him with both human and material resources.

What seemed to be fundamental was the service's ability to provide an immediate response to the needs which emerged in this situation. It saw these needs as urgent not because of some potential danger but because it recognized that a need, once expressed, is always urgent. In this period A.'s delirious core seemed to waste away and disappear from his expressions and emotions.

On 16 January 1984 three workers from the centre went with A. for the final revoking of security measures. A. would now no longer have to return to the JPH.

Part II

Policy, Power and Changing Roles

Editor's Introduction

The contributions to this section focus on the objectives of a real change in the psychiatric systems and on the processes by which such change can be achieved.

There is a broad agreement that the aim of restructuring psychiatry is to give a new status to users, new roles for the workers and to achieve new attitudes by the public (Kingsley and Towell). However, the specific meaning given to the 'newness' within these three components differs not only between the Italian and the British but also within the British camp: thus the Exeter experience is about the closure of the hospitals and the construction of local services (Chapter 17), while the Chesterfield project is much more concerned with putting into practice the principle of empowering users (Chapter 19).

More of the differences between the British and Italian ways of thinking about psychiatry and effecting change in the system come to the fore in this part than in Part I. The differences seem to be centred on what is fundamentally wrong with traditional psychiatry and which are the most important steps required in order to effect a real change in it. (See in particular Chapters 15, 16, 17, 18, 23 and 24).

Both sides are aware and weary of the risk of 'trans-institutionalism', or the mere transfer of people from one institutional setting (the hospital) to another (located outside the hospital), dressed as 'community care'. However, the Italians are stressing the need for a drastic change inside the psychiatric hospital as a precondition to secure a real change in the psychiatric services to be offered outside. This need is in part seen as a means to break down the barrier of silence, denial and expulsion which typified the public's approach to mental illness and which has been internalized by both patients and staff to varying degrees (see Rotelli, Del Giudice, De Nicola and Basaglia). In part, the powerful process of changing the arch-psychiatric institution (i.e. the hospital) is perceived as a very powerful tool in changing the staff's, patients', public's attitudes to and knowledge of mental distress.

It is perhaps due to the newness of the very possibility of the closure of hospitals in Britain that the British contributions do not in fact focus much on the process of the closure, but on the 'life after', namely the psychiatric community service. In addition, the separation of health and social services in the UK seems to be leading to thinking in terms of specializing services located in one or the other sector, rather than what are the overall needs in terms of services. This issue remains as a major area which requires close attention, conceptual and practical development in the UK.

The comparison between the comprehensiveness of the Italian community mental health centres (see Chapters 18 and 20) and the specificity of a mental health resource centre or the Exeter local services (Chapters 19 and 17) illustrates this aspect.

The focal point of Part II is the required change in the attitudes and skills of professionals and the processes of achieving these changes. These attitudes and skills are closely connected to the relationships which the workers have with other components of the psychiatric system and their place in society; hence this focus mirrors the whole transformation of the psychiatric system.

De Nicola, Giacobbi and Rogialli (Chapter 22) describe with candour professional practices in the hospital of the past compared to those in the present changed system, concluding that the satisfaction of moving from a custodial to an informal therapeutic role is a primary motivation for change, which needs to be encouraged. King (Chapter 17) stresses the need to secure a non-redundancy policy and a dialogue with the trade unions if workers are not to be initially threatened by the transition. Hennelly (Chapter 19) demonstrates some of the new possibilities and problems which exist when workers move to become background enablers in the process of empowering users. The MIND Manchester group (Chapter 21) focuses on the real sense of powerlessness of those workers who would like to see their setting changed but feel isolated by those who actively object to change: let us remember that the more real the change becomes, the stronger the resistance to it, based as it is on years of training, on fear of loss of power and the belief in the preference of the clinical-somatic approach to mental distress. These elements have been convincingly exposed by Bourne and Basaglia in Chapters 23 and 24, despite the disagreement of these two authors on the value of medicine as we know it.

Some of the issues 'forgotten' in Part I surface in this section, namely living in a hostile work climate (Manchester MIND, Hennelly, De Nicola, Del Giudice), relatives of direct users (Losavio, MIND group), privatization (Losavio) and cost (Kingsley and Towell, Rotelli, King). The issue of cost is related to the context of welfare policies and the changing approaches to state initiated welfare services, which are commented upon both in Part I and in Chapters 15 and 16. We need to ask ourselves whether and how, with the reappraisal of the welfare state, we may have the opportunity to undo the harm of some of its components (see Chapters 23 and 24), as well as retaining its positive elements.

Above all, the contributions to this section demonstrate not only that the psychiatric system needs to be changed at its core, but that it is possible, useful and satisfying to do so, despite the endless difficulties encountered in the process. Rotelli summarizes neatly the essence of this exercise: it is about investing in people, not in settings.

Shulamit Ramon

15
Changing Psychiatric Services in Britain

DAVID TOWELL, SU KINGSLEY

In Britain as in many other countries, the period since the Second World War has seen significant changes in psychiatric practice, the general trend of which has been the shift away from the Victorian inheritance of institutional provision towards a more community-based pattern of services. National policies promoting these changes have not, however, evolved in a single, coherent way. Nor have they been implemented uniformly. Reform in psychiatric services necessarily emerges from the complex interplay of bureaucratic, professional and community pressures, within the wider economic, social and political context.[1] In devising strategies appropriate to developing psychiatric services in the next decade, it is important that lessons are learnt from earlier experience.[2]

Two examples will suffice to introduce the major themes of this chapter. The immediate post-war years saw Britain with a socialist government committed to major social reconstruction. Its large majority reflected a popular mandate for radical change, including introduction of the welfare state and with it, creation of the NHS. The mental hospitals were incorporated into the NHS and though most were slow to benefit, there was a scatter of institutions, typically with young doctors back from military service in leadership positions, where an early start was made on a programme of liberalization. Wards were unlocked, custodial attitudes challenged, meaningful work provided for patients, links established with the developing community health services and rehabilitation actively pursued. These changes were carried further in some places through the development of the therapeutic community philosophy with its stress on democratization and open communication. The doctors became administrative therapists and Britain led the European movement towards Social Psychiatry.[3]

These innovations took time to generalize and 20 years on were still being introduced in some places. By the mid-1960s however the movement for reform had changed in significant ways. The 1959 Mental Health Act gave legal expression to some liberalization in the status of mental patients but the psychotropic drugs were commonly given much of the credit for previous achievements. There was again a Labour government, this time aiming to harness new technology to secure its expansionary economic and social goals. In the NHS there was expensive investment in district general hospitals and psychiatric units were gradually incorporated into these centres of high technology medicine. Further reform in psychiatry was seen as achievable through the integration of acute provision for mental and physical illness and it was hoped that such integration would also bring new public attitudes to psychiatric disabilities. The administrative therapists again became proper doctors and the therapeutic community approach declined in influence.[4]

Now, another 20 years on, the situation of British psychiatry reflects this history. The emphasis on rehabilitation and the shift of acute services have led to a large reduction in the occupancy of mental hospitals – a reduction which would have been much more dramatic but for the inappropriate admission of confused elderly people, turning many institutions into huge old people's homes. After a century or more of use, the physical condition of the original asylums is declining and they are increasingly costly to maintain. There are again significant pressures for change, focusing on closure of the institutions and the use of their resources to develop local alternatives.

Past failure to integrate different aspects of reform and to sustain the momentum for change means that in 1986 the implementation of good community-based mental health services still constitutes a major challenge. Moreover progress must be sought under conditions which are quite different from those of earlier reforms. A strong right-wing government is committed to cutting public expenditure, and its social policies offer little support for liberal attitudes or concern with the disadvantaged. Much of the current impetus for change derives from the NHS bureaucracy and its preoccupation with more efficient use of resources tied up in the mental hospitals. The vision of alternative provision is poorly defined however and there is considerable danger that rather than developing new services, the relocation of resources will merely reproduce old services in new places.

In our view the scale of this challenge has been underestimated. Real change in psychiatric provision will only be attained where it is possible to achieve new status for people with psychiatric disabilities, new roles for staff and new public attitudes all within a single movement for reform.

We cannot be sanguine about the prospects for success in the next few years. From what is already happening, often on a small scale, in different parts of Britain,[5] we are convinced however that even within the existing climate and framework for public services, there are significant opportunities to make progress. Focusing particularly on the pattern of mental health services required to support people with severe psychiatric disabilities, the remainder of this chapter examines the practical strategies required to make good use of these opportunities.

Elements in Strategies for Purposeful Change

Our analysis suggests that successful strategies for developing community-based psychiatric services have two fundamental requirements: change should be *principled* and change should be *systemic*.

Defining Service Principles

In arguing for principled change, our concern is to overcome the weaknesses in provision which can be expected if the combination of ill-defined national policies, professional conservatism and traditional pragmatism allows present assumptions to colonize the future. Instead it is vitally important that change should be guided by explicit principles which make clear how new services will enhance the life experiences of people with particular psychiatric disabilities. This is especially the case in considering the futures available to people requiring help on a long-term basis, who may be most at risk of being devalued and have certainly suffered from inadequate services in the past.

As the MIND manifesto *Common Concern*[6] argues more fully, explicit service principles provide the foundation both for service design and subsequent quality assurance. The definition of these principles needs to address two sets of questions: the first concerned with effectiveness and acceptability of services to individual users; the second concerned with accessibility of services and their relevance to needs of the local population. In the former category, we believe these principles should stress the importance of guaranteeing the rights, maintaining the dignity and avoiding stigmatization of people with severe psychiatric disabilities. They should also underline the objective of providing services which support people in living their lives as far as possible in ordinary neighbourhoods and minimizing their handicaps. In the latter category, important aims should include providing services which are comprehensive – through offering a range of support to everyone in the local population with severe disabilities, and appropriate – through recognizing variations in need among different users.[7]

Addressing the Total System of Psychiatric Provision
In arguing for systemic change, we aim to draw attention, first, to the complex organization of major public agencies and their interactions with the people and communities they serve; and second, to the variety of interest groups necessarily affected by the transition to new patterns of provision. The questions for reformers are:

- How can a coalition in support of principled change be assembled?
- What activities will be required to secure implementation of local services based on these principles?

In examining the current organization of relevant services in Britain, we have found it useful to distinguish three main components of systemic change:

- Establishing the strategic framework;
- Managing existing services, particularly the contracting mental hospitals;
- Developing community-based services.

Table 15.1 on p. 174 illustrates the interdependence of these three components and lists key issues which need to be addressed in planning action. Our discussion of these issues seeks to identify lessons from British experience about how best to achieve purposeful change.

Establishing the Strategic Framework
As we noted earlier, in contrast with other periods of reform, the main thrust behind current plans to relocate resources from the institutions stems from government and regional authorities and their quest for efficiency.[8] As with other bureaucratic reforms, it is all too easy in this situation for mental hospital staff and patients to see themselves as victims of change rather than active participants in creating community-based psychiatric provision. While impetus from government and regions may be important in sustaining the momentum for change, new patterns of services cannot be achieved solely by 'top down' planning and mechanistic control. Our own work with authorities in different parts of the country has shown that real change in services at the point where people with psychiatric disabilities and front-line staff meet requires strong local leadership and mobilization of widespread participation in an organic process of development.[9]

In the past psychiatric services and their users have not been given consistent priority in the contest with more 'popular' causes and acute

Table 15.1 Key Issues in a Concerted Strategy for Change

Establishing the Strategic Framework

Strategic		
		policy leadership
		political backing
		vision and principles
		management arrangements
		financial policies
		personnel policies
		support for innovation and staff training

	Managing Contracting Institutions	Developing Local Services
	co-ordination arrangements	establishing shared visions
	staff consultation and participation	joint planning processes
	redeployment policies	participative planning
	retrenchment strategy	individual needs
	maintaining quality and morals	staff training
	individual patient relocation	innovation, evaluation, quality assurance

Operational		
	Large Hospitals	Local Services

medical specialities. Given the magnitude and duration of the transition towards local services, progress is only likely to be maintained where efforts are made to build explicit political support for reform – represented, for example, in the interest and commitment of local and health authority members. As experience in the South East Thames region has demonstrated,[10] this political support is particularly important in ensuring that the necessary resources are made available both to fund local services and meet the extra costs involved in transition.

There is no doubt that the substantial assets of money and skill tied up in the old institutions can be used more effectively in providing community-based alternatives. Given the poor quality of past provision however, experiences in Exeter, Riverside and the North East Thames region suggest that the total public sector cost of acceptable new services is likely to be greater than current expenditure – although drawn from a wider range of sources, including significant increases from the social security budget. During the transition period there is also a need for 'bridging' finance to create the infrastructure for new services and meet the increasingly expensive unit costs of the contracting institutions before their total replacement.[11]

Bringing these points together, it follows that the task of government and regional agencies is to establish a broad strategic framework designed to encourage local leadership and provide incentives for decentralized service development. Among the issues this framework will need to address are the rate of change towards community-based services, the financial policies required to offer incentives for local innovation while protecting standards in the contracting institutions, and the personnel and training policies necessary to foster staff commitment to change and ensure that appropriately skilled people are available to provide new services.

It is also important that this strategic framework is based on recognition that support to people with psychiatric disabilities should in future draw upon the contribution of several different public agencies, including the NHS, local authority social services, housing, education and leisure provision, employment services, and social security offices, as well as from the voluntary sector. In the past these services have often been fragmented and there is no doubt that co-ordinating development across the multiplicity of agencies in each large hospital catchment area is a complex organizational challenge. Nevertheless significant change is unlikely to be successful unless the main agencies work together in planning and implementation. Our own research has shown that the creation of joint fora and wider networks which address the total system of psychiatric service provision are essential mechanisms for coping with this complexity.[12]

Managing Existing Services

A central component of the current service system is of course the mental hospitals whose position and contribution require careful attention during the period of transition. There are two possible risks here. One is that existing institutional concerns will dominate local planning and seriously handicap the fresh thinking required to create community-based alternatives. The other is that the mental hospitals will be excluded from planning for the future and their staff left to struggle with the consequences of development elsewhere. Both these risks can be avoided however if relevant parts of the mental hospitals are represented in the local planning and co-ordination arrangements established to ensure the successful relocation and rehabilitation of present in-patients.

At the same time it is vital to recognize that management of the institutions during a lengthy period of contraction is itself a major task. The mental hospitals continue to need high quality management committed to involving staff in maintaining and where possible improving standards while relocation is proceeding.

A significant weakness in many British initiatives for change however has been the belated attention given to securing the support of existing staff, the majority of whom still work in the mental hospitals. It is to be expected that staff interests may be mobilized to protect the status quo, particularly at a time of mass únemployment, unless from the outset personnel and training policies are negotiated which seek to maximize continuity of employment. Neither the maintenance of standards in the contracting hospitals nor appropriate preparation for patients moving to local services is likely unless efforts have been made to gain the support of existing staff for change.[13] How this can be done is again well illustrated by experience in Exeter and Riverside.[14]

Developing Community-based Services

New patterns of local services can only be created where traditional bureaucratic approaches to planning and implementation are replaced by an organic process of service development which promotes widespread participation in achieving change on the basis of explicit values and principles. We have already argued the importance of a principled approach to change. As people in north Lincolnshire have demonstrated,[15] it is at local level that all the legitimate interests (people with psychiatric disabilities, the public, professional groups and representatives of the service-providing agencies) can be engaged in the debate necessary both to shape and gain commitment to a new vision of future provision. An essential task of local leadership is to ensure this debate starts from the experiences of people with psychiatric disabilities. On this basis, the new Social Psychiatry will be just as concerned with promoting their status and participation in the wider community through attention to income, homes and jobs as with specific interventions to reduce handicaps and encourage personal development.

In the past, particularly where planning has addressed the requirements of large populations, client needs have been aggregated into ill-defined categories which fail to reflect individual diversity. There has also been a tendency to concentrate on people's disabilities rather than their abilities and to define needs in terms of the way services are currently provided rather than functionally, by the assistance actually required. The resulting services have often been agency- rather than client-centred. The new approach to planning begins instead from a careful assessment of individual strengths, needs and wishes and seeks to deliver services which meet changing individual requirements.[16]

It follows of course that local planning must involve people with psychiatric disabilities themselves, where necessary establishing independent sources of advice and representation to strengthen the consumers' voice in service development. For example, staff from Friern Hospital and Camden Social Services have shown that for patients currently living in the mental hospitals this may involve local project teams in intensive 'getting to know you' exercises which make the person's own experiences central to identifying his or her future requirements.[17] The development of outreach services from generic Citizens Advice Bureaux and more specific one-to-one advocacy schemes are two possible ways of offering patients independent support, as well as assisting their access to services like social security.[18] This concern to plan on the basis of client needs and wishes must also include people with psychiatric disabilities already living in the community, whether or not they are regular users of existing specialist services.

The development of genuinely community-based services cannot of course be achieved solely by welfare agencies and their professional employees: rather, the participative approach to planning must seek to foster partnership between community services and the community itself, both to gain public support for new patterns of local services and in the longer term to promote fuller integration of people with psychiatric disabilities in community life. Appreciating individual client needs, developing services which are responsive to local differences, for example in demography and ethnicity, and building this partnership are all more likely where planning for the populations of large administrative areas (health districts, boroughs etc.) starts by addressing the requirements of small localities, as the wider experiments in decentralizing public services are demonstrating.[19]

In the context of these several aspects of innovative planning, new patterns of services can be designed. Essentially, service design involves assessing how well alternative models of provision meet individual needs and are consistent with agreed principles. Typically a range of alternatives should be considered, drawn from promising experience elsewhere (like that documented in other chapters of this book)[20] and from local invention.

Again, as the Exeter experience suggests, this creative process of local service development must however go beyond planning to ensure that good intentions are realized in practice and high quality services are maintained and improved in the light of experience. First, this involves ensuring that planning and implementation are closely linked: staff who are to lead service delivery should be involved in planning these services; service design should be expressed in detailed operational policies and management arrangements; and all staff should be trained in the procedures required to put these policies into practice. Second, this requires that local services should build in explicit arrangements for quality assurance, again starting from the principles upon which services have been based.

Finally, running through these local development processes and growing from the shared experience of new forms of service provision, there will need to be a major effort to clarify the values, concepts and personal skills required to underpin the practice of community-based psychiatry (as later chapters of this book argue more fully).

Energizing Reform

To return to our starting point however, these prescriptions for incremental reform must be related to the wider context. Britain's continuing economic decline and the influential political ideologies which devalue public services and seek to stretch further the informal caring contribution of families are a major handicap to the modest aspirations which we have described. There are real dangers for vulnerable people that change in this climate will at best result in 'trans-institutionalization' and at worst add to their poverty and neglect.[21]

While recognizing these dangers, our position is that people with severe psychiatric disabilities cannot wait for more desirable economic and political conditions. More positively, our analysis of the best of what is already being achieved in different parts of the country suggests that real opportunities are available even in current circumstances to make progress in enhancing the status and support for people with psychiatric disabilities in their own communities.

We appreciate the scale of the challenge. The British welfare state is the largest and most complex bureaucratic organization in Europe. To use its strength as a vehicle for addressing individual need in a community context will require inspiration, commitment and ingenuity. We have summarized what we believe should be elements in the movement for reform. Most important among these is the need for local people to reclaim the leadership for change – mobilizing active coalitions of relevant interests (including consumers, community representatives, progressive staff, managers and policy-makers) around a vision of future services which is rooted in the experience of people with psychiatric disabilities and reflects their entitlement to something better.

We believe such leadership can link further reform of psychiatric provision to the wider values already visible in early post-war achievements and still reflected in popular support for the welfare state. In particular, the concepts of *citizenship* and *community*, suitably updated to reflect the social conditions now prevailing, have continuing appeal. For people with psychiatric disabilities, citizenship implies the right to participate in economic, social and cultural life and to receive the support necessary to make this possible – decent housing, income, work opportunities and professional help when required. The idea of community suggests that these rights can only be realized through a partnership between public services and ordinary people. The fuller participation of people with disabilities would constitute a community achievement: reflecting the community's commitment to accepting all its members and developing all its human resources.

In conclusion we should emphasize again that our expectations for the benefits of psychiatric reform are modest. While community mental health should benefit from collective action designed to secure wider social change, we remain doubtful about the converse proposition: that society itself can be changed through initiatives addressed primarily to people already suffering major disadvantage.[22] In making some gains for and with this vulnerable group of people however, what we *learn* may well have rather wider relevance. We may see more clearly what would be involved in achieving citizenship and community for us all.

References

1. The government White Paper (1975) *Better Services for the Mentally Ill*, HMSO, London, Cmnd. 6233, provides the fullest official expression of this trend, although national policies were restated in the DHSS paper (1985) 'Mental Illness: Policies For Prevention, Treatment, Rehabilitation And Care' in *Government Response to the Social Services Committee*, 1984–5 Session Cmnd. 9674, HMSO, London. They were given added impetus through the financial mechanisms of the *Care in the Community* initiative (DHSS *Health Service Development: Care in the Community and Joint Finance* HC(83)6 LAC(83)5) and legislative changes which define the rights of individuals requiring treatment. See Gostin, L. (1983) *A Practical Guide to Mental Health Law*, MIND, London.

2. For further historical analysis, see for example, Ramon, S. (1985) *Psychiatry in Britain*, Croom Helm, London.

3. Discussed further in Clark, D.H. (1981) *Social Therapy in Psychiatry*, Churchill Livingstone, London.

4. Contemporary studies include: Hoenig, J., Hamilton, M.W. (1969) *The De-Segregation of the Mentally Ill*, Routledge & Kegan Paul, London; Baruch, G., Treacher, A. (1978) *Psychiatry Observed*, Routledge & Kegan Paul, London; and Towell, D. (1975) *Understanding Psychiatric Nursing*, Royal College of Nursing, London.

5. For a detailed review, see Towell D., McAusland T. (eds) 'Managing Psychiatric Services in Transition', *Health and Social Service Journal*, 18 October 1984.

6. *Common Concern: MIND's Manifesto for a New Mental Health Service* (1983) MIND, London.

7. Good examples of well-designed local services based on explicit principles, in this case relating to ordinary housing for people with major long-term disabilities, can be found in the GPMH *Housing Information Pack* (1985) GPMH, London.

8. An analysis of Regional Health Authority strategies is presented in MIND's *Common Concern*.

9. See for further discussion Towell, D., Harries C.J. (eds) (1979) *Innovation in Patient Care*, Croom Helm, London.

10. See Korman, N., Glennerster, H. (1985) *Closing a Hospital*, Bedford Square Press, London.

11. These financial issues are discussed further in Towell, D., McAusland, T. *Psychiatric Services*. Detailed cost projections have been prepared by a number of health authorities, notably Riverside DHA.

12. See, for example, Towell, D., 'Developing Better Services for the Mentally Ill' in Barrett, S., Fudge, C. (eds) (1981) *Policy and Action*, Methuen, London.

13. Issues elaborated in Towell, D., Davis, A. (1984) 'Moving out from the Large Hospitals: Involving the people (staff and patients) concerned', *Care in the Community – Keeping It Local*, MIND, London.

14. See the contributions by King, D., Colclough, P., Dexter, M., Foley, B., in Towell, D. and McAusland T., *Psychiatric Services*.

15. See for details, Collin, A.J. (1985) 'Transition in Mental Illness Services – Creativitiy in Planning', *Hospital and Health Services Review*, 'September, pp. 235–7.

16. A model for implementing this approach in relation to existing hospital in-patients has been developed in our work with Claybury Hospital. See McAusland, T., Towell, D., Kinsley, S. (1986) *Assessment, Resettlement and Rehabilitation: Designing the arrangements for moving people from*

psychiatric hospitals into local services, King's Fund College, London.

17. Described by Braisby, D. 'On the road to self-reliance', *Social Work Today,* 6 August, pp. 16–17.

18. See for example, Davis, A., Hayton, C. (1984) *Who Benefits?* Birmingham University Department of Social Administration; and *Inside Advice* (1985) Tooting Bec Hospital Citizens Advice Bureau, London.

19. One approach is described by King, D., Court, M. (1984) 'A sense of scale: the shift to locality planning', *Health and Social Service Journal,* 21 June, p. 734.

20. One useful European compilation is *Alternatives to Mental Hospitals* (1980) MIND/IHF, London. An information service on innovative local projects is provided by Good Practices in Mental Health, 380 Harrow Road, London W9 2HU.

21. See, for example, House of Commons (1985) *Second Report from the Social Services Committee, Session 1984–5: Community Care with Special Reference to Adult Mentally Ill and Mentally Handicapped People* HMSO, London.

22. For discussion of a more radical position, see Banton, R. et al. (1985) *The Politics of Mental Health,* Macmillan, London.

16

Changing Psychiatric Services in Italy

FRANCO ROTELLI

The great period of reform which in the last 20 years involved and sometimes transformed to varying degrees mental health systems in Europe and the US, was spearheaded by the intention to renew the therapeutic capacity of psychiatry. This it intended to do by freeing itself from the archaic function as an instrument of social control, coercion and segregation. In this political and cultural context, de-institutionalization was a central watchword used for many different ends: for 'reformers' it in fact summed up the objectives; for 'radical' groups of professionals and politicians it symbolized the prospect of abolishing all social control institutions and aligned itself with the anti-psychiatric point of view. For administrators it was primarily a programme of financial and administrative rationalization. This meant a reduction in hospital beds, one of the first tasks to be undertaken in the wake of the fiscal crisis.

De-institutionalization has in fact taken place according to the last definition. That is, it has been put into practice by de-hospitalizing patients and by a gradual reduction in the number of beds; in some cases, by closing psychiatric hospitals quite abruptly.

Innovative Italian psychiatrists work on the hypothesis that the hidden fault of psychiatry is having separated a fictitious object, the 'illness', from the overall existence of users and from the body of society. A whole body of scientific, legislative and administrative apparatus ('the institution') has been built on this artificial separation. It is this body which must be dismantled ('de-institutionalization') in order to re-establish contact with users' lives in so far as they are 'sick lives'.

The radical nature of this critique about what psychiatry really is and its role in the larger social system does not mean that innovative psychiatrists embark upon the anti-psychiatry short cut. The route which they take is more complex and indirect. Along this way, the therapeutic objective and task is firmly monitored (therefore we are not politicizing), yet at the same time the power (residual, but irreplaceable) which psychiatry holds in the institutional system is used as the power for reform: therefore we are politicizing.

The first step for de-institutionalization has been to begin dismantling the problem–solution relationship. This can be achieved by no longer aspiring to the radical solution (which is potentially optimization) of fully restoring normality. This certainly does not mean forgoing the possibility of a cure. This sort of 'relinquishing' belongs to the family of so-called 'indirect strategies' which regards objectives such as health as achievable only as by-products. Deferring the solution sets off a profound and enduring change of perspective which pervades the whole of institutional actions and interactions.

From direct observation of the mental hospital (and is this not so for the general hospital also?) it is evident that in the relationship between problem and solution, it is the solution which formulates the problem. This is why the first step towards de-institutionalization must be to no longer emphasize classification of a particular illness but to concentrate instead on a practical approach. In fact any attempt at explaining the causes should be abandoned. This must go beyond the chain of standard diagnoses, scientific definitions and institutional structures through which mental illness – i.e. the problem – has assumed these forms of existence and expression.[1] For this reason, deferring the solution completely changes the therapeutic action into action for institutional change.

For example, in the process leading to the closure of the psychiatric hospital in Trieste, we initially focused on groups of residents changing their style of life inside the institution. We deliberately did not focus on attention to individuals, on assessing their abilities and needs in the oppressive institution, or on moving them outside the hospital. Only when we thought that their lifestyle – and that of the institution – had changed sufficiently to resemble ordinary life, did we start to encourage them to think about moving out.

We can say therefore that de-institutionalization is practical work aimed at change, starting with the mental hospital. It takes apart the existing institutional solution in order to dismantle, and then reconstitute, the problem. In other words, the ways in which people are cured (or not cured) are changed in order *to change their suffering*.

By breaking the clinical model, the central role of modern, real welfare services can be interpreted as *the institutional multipliers of energy*. The process of de-institutionalization therefore becomes a reconstruction of the object's complexity. Emphasis is no longer placed on the healing process but on a plan for creating health and social reproduction.

The work of dismantling the mental hospital from the inside uncovers several crucial aspects. These contribute to a greater understanding of the meaning of Italian de-institutionalization and the ways in which it took place.

How De-institutionalization Mobilizes all Participants Involved in the System of Institutional Action

As Chapter 18 describes, we had several long, daily meetings. Some of these were for everyone, while others were for residents mainly or primarily for the staff. They became the main tool for attitudinal change of both the workers and the residents. The principal actors in the de-institutionalization process are primarily the professionals who work in the institutions. It is they who change the organization, the relationships and the rules of the game by actively carrying out the therapeutic roles of psychiatrist, nurse, psychologist etc. On this basis patients too become actors. The therapeutic relationship becomes a source of power which can be used to remind them of responsibility and power, of other institutional actors, of local administrators responsible for mental health, of professionals in local health structures and of politicians. In other words mental health professionals activate the entire network of relationships which the system of institutional action is built on including all the specialisms' powers, interests and social requirements. This is why they too are indirectly politicizing. But only indirectly, since they remain linked to their profession. This is their source of power and a condition for directly practising the objectives for change.

This is an important aspect of Italian de-institutionalization, and one which distinguishes it from other experiences – i.e. it was planned by reforming professionals, applied by administrators or proclaimed as a political objective by radical groups and movements. It took place as practical, professional, everyday work which gradually produced changes. The new politics of mental health were constructed on a practical, local basis from within the institution, where even politics was used as a medium or resource. This is why society at large finds itself caught up, involved in and mobilized as actors in the change: patients, the local community, public opinion and politicians. Thus with the support of local artists we have prepared a show, open to everyone, and as part of which we went in a procession into the centre of the town. The centrepiece of the procession was a blue horse, made by all of us, symbolizing the force we were liberating from invisibility. This way of implementing de-institutionalization inspires and multiplies relationships; it produces communication, solidarity and conflict because structural change can only take place alongside a change in society and its culture.

Why the Prime Objective of De-institutionalization is to Transform Power Relationships between the Institution and its Patients

At the beginning of work for dismantling the mental hospital this change is produced by simple alterations: eliminating the means of containment, renewing the individual's relationship with his body, giving back to him/her the right and the ability to use personal objects, giving back to him/her the right to and the ability for verbal expression, eliminating occupational therapy, opening doors, producing relationships, space and topics of conversation, freeing emotions, reinstating civil rights, and eliminating coercion, judicial custody and 'the land of danger', and reactivating a revenue base to gain access to social exchanges.

These are only simple changes and are fairly well known. But we are restating them here for two reasons. Firstly, because our direct knowledge of reformed psychiatric internment establishments in Europe today, and our analyses of the regulations governing them, tell us that these changes have yet to be implemented. Secondly, because the simplicity of these changes helps to understand how de-institutionalization is primarily therapeutic work, aimed at putting individuals back together again regardless of their illness. When 'the healing solution' is put to one side it can be seen that caring means acting here and now to change a patient's way of life and experiencing his/her pain and to change the life which his/her suffering feeds on in practical, everyday terms.

Psychiatric illness is unlikely to disappear, but one will begin to remove the reasons for it. The ways and the importance which the illness assumes in a person's life will change. But the person's need for help and care will still remain. We will be reminded of the value of these needs and the need for patients to be valued.

For example, this means that one does not give psychiatric patients work as a result of, or in recognition of, an improvement in their condition (a reward), nor as therapy, but as a preliminary requisite for their improvement – a right.[2] This component was developed so as to avoid leaving the patient to his/her own devices (in the name of some abstract concept of freedom). Yet it attempts to avoid imposing predetermined objectives on him/her.

The change in the power relationship between patients and the institution is a process which takes place on a large scale and must involve the legal system. Right up until Law 180 was passed in 1978, those who were conducting experiments in de-institutionalization paid obsessive attention to:

- gradually making new laws more impartial;
- and to ensuring they were recognized first by the administration and then by the judiciary.

In fact de-institutionalization gradually changes a patient's legal status (from compulsory patient to voluntary patient, then from patient to 'guest', then to the elimination of all types of custody and afterwards to the restoration of all civil rights). The patient becomes a citizen with full rights and the nature of his/her agreement with the various services changes. In this sense therapeutic work provides an example to sociological literature about relationships between actor and system and on the conditions of social change.

De-institutionalization as Homeopathic Work which uses the Internal Energies of the Institution to Dismantle Itself

Changes in the institution are brought about from the inside by working on what is there. De-institutionalization of the mental hospital uses the same spaces, the same resources, the same staff and the same patients. However, it changes and separates the systems of action and interaction in which each element is inserted: a door made to be closed is used actively by opening it. This act creates problems. Managing these problems changes the culture of the participants in question. Again, we see the fundamental difference between the Italian mode of de-institutionalization and others: it is based on using resources and problems *inside the structure* which is being dismantled in order to build *new external structures* piece by piece. These structures are created so that patients can gradually be accompanied outside the mental hospital, and so that alternatives and the necessary culture can be built: district services, psychiatric night duty in general hospitals, co-operatives, houses for ex-patients, bars, area canteens, gymnasiums, theatre workshops etc.

In other words the structures and working practices which the new mental health system is based on, are created by gradually recycling, converting, and transforming financial facilities, personnel and existing authorities and functions. They are not created from the outside or alongside and in addition to the mental hsopital. It is precisely because they are created by dismantling the mental hospital that they succeed in *replacing it completely* and in suppressing former procedures.

To sum up, the process of de-institutionalization is characterized by these three aspects which gradually take shape as the mental hospital is disbanded. They also represent its basic features:

- *Construction of a new mental health policy* from the bottom up and from within institutional structures. This is achieved by the mobilization and participation (even conflicting participation) of all the interested parties;
- *The aim of enriching patients' overall existence must be central to therapeutic work*. In this way patients (both severely and slightly ill) are active subjects and not objects in their relationship with the institutions. The watchword is: from the mental hospital as a place where even social exchanges were non-existent to the obverse of actual, multiple social relationships.
- *The creation of external structures which totally replace internment in a mental hospital*: precisely because they arise from the inside, out of its dismantling and by using and changing its material and human resources.

These three aspects of de-institutionalization provide conditions which favour the exclusion of internment from combined psychiatric structures and authority. Or to be more precise it can be said that by taking this route de-institutionalization abolishes internment and frees psychiatry and its object (and ultimately society) from the *need* for internment. It changes the needs of sick people, workers and the community to which internment provided a response by constructing entirely different responses.

Changing the Ways of Administering Public Resources for Mental Health

As we have already said, dismantling the mental hospital has taken place by using and changing existing resources. New facilities take shape with the physical removal of staff, patients, and funds from the hospital to the community. The changing financial and administrative management of public resources benefits from new effectiveness and efficiency.

The basic point is that the local administration no longer uses available resources for providing an institutional structure – the hospital. This type of structure essentially measures its costs according to the cost of board and lodging for each bed and their optimum use is based on maximizing the number of beds occupied. Instead these resources are used for providing direct services to the individuals concerned based on the following criteria:

- *Mobility of staff* in the physical sense, since patients no longer go to the service but the service goes to the users;
- *Individuality of the service*, i.e. the quantity and quality of resources supplied is commensurate with the needs of individual patients and varies with those needs;
- *Increase of resources managed directly by clients* and which are more directly concerned with their lives (see the reduction of expenditure on drugs and the increase on sickness benefit demonstrated between 1970 and 1980 in Trieste);[3]
- *Productive use of resources*, i.e. increased expenditure in financing users' work which is socially useful (for instance, grants or financial contributions to co-operatives);
- *Increasing use of resources activated and organized by associations between ex-patients and the community*, or by associations between users themselves; this also means promoting and protecting self-help and autonomous groups.

These criteria are primarily designed to increase therapeutic effectiveness. This effectiveness can be evaluated by taking into consideration that the system does not offer selection and exclusion, but is capable of avoiding and reversing processes whereby certain needs become chronic. The most obvious indication for evaluating the effectiveness of this system is that it does not perpetuate the need for internment.

Administering public resources in this way also rationalizes expenditure. Waste and automatic fixed costs and expenses which usually overwhelm bureaucratic organizations are reduced. All things considered, the new system does not cost more. This is important, especially in times of public expenditure cuts. However, this is an indirect benefit of a system which aims to invest resources in people (and possibly increase resources) rather than in institutions.

If 'freedom is therapeutic', any act of freedom can be therapeutic. If the de-institutionalization of illness is considered an experience which cannot be separated from life, the combination of positive resources from the service and its users must be valued more than the symptoms of illness (upon which institutions are built). Of course, an enormous range of professional skills is required by this type of practice. Therapeutic work must involve a complex field of action:

- For example, though the accepted code of practice in medicine and its services seems to be elimination of the *emotional dimension*, in this case the emotional dimension has value.

- Though it may be accepted practice to separate the setting in which professionals and users interact from the wider context, in this instance every possible way of placing the relationship in the wider context is sought.
- Though the presence of non-professional figures in the medical field is usually viewed with suspicion, every effort is made here to introduce non-professionals into the service to act as critical, de-institutionalizing factors. These include local priests and church people, local political parties and local artists.
- Though regulations in a service are usually welcome, here they tend to be regarded as *detrimental to the promotion of social and therapeutic exchanges* and are criticized and removed wherever possible.
- Though health services are usually very separate, every effort should be made to ensure that they are accessible and used by the local people.
- Though the relationship with the 'illness' is always referred to a hospital, clinic etc. de-institutionalization requires a relationship with the neighbourhood.
- Finally, de-institutionalization cannot take place by separating acute cases from chronic cases, otherwise the criteria for mixing people would still be their type of 'illness' (and therefore chronic cases would be created again, making the service ineffective). Instead all applications must be met initially in the same way.

All of this is de-institutionalization. It is a complex task for workers and administrators. However, it does allow essential participation in community resources and enormous potential for mobilizing energy.

Emphasis on de-institutionalization is linked also to an economic plan. This plan regards the old general organization of psychiatric institutions as backward and wasteful. Users of these institutions are deprived of their energies and resourcefulness and often this deprivation becomes the aim of these institutions.

From all this, it can be seen that de-institutionalization as it is understood by *Psichiatria Democratica* (PD), is the exact opposite of all types of neglect. Where I work, the economic and human resources which were used by one large psychiatric hospital in 1971 are all used in the community, and by the community, as Chapter 18 describes.[4]

Conclusion

De-institutionalization is the process of eliminating all the violent simplifications which were traditionally operated by psychiatry. It means rediscovering the complexity of psychiatry's object. It is a way of leaving behind the asylum model and the grey deductive ambiguities of the clinical and the psychological models.

De-institutionalization offered a way forward after the institutional problems which had been highlighted by the fiscal crisis and the critics of waste and bureaucracy. It showed how the production crisis could be used to increase effectiveness. The experiment of dismantling mental hospitals had already shown that this too was an ineffective institutional response concerning mental health needs. It also served to demonstrate that qualitative change of existing resources was not only possible but also more effective. In other words, as has already been mentioned, *much less investment in apparatus and more in people,* less for maintaining institutions and their bureaucracies and more for maintaining people's autonomy.

De-institutionalization, which arose out of the social reforms in the welfare years, highlights the effects of policies which have been handed from the top down rather than by evolving from the bottom up. These are effects on people who have been reformed by the social services and who have had responsibility taken away from them by the institution, and are now fully dependent on it. Let us assume that these are not the effects of welfare but of that particular type of welfare. New mental health policy is a field where *cultures of need and resources* are developed; where people, local communities and users organize themselves for action, develop solutions and introduce changes to the functioning of institutional structures.

References

1. Basaglia, F. (1968) *L'Istituzione Negata*, Einaudi, Milan.
2. Mauri, D. et al. (1983) *La Libertà è Terapeutica?* Feltrinelli, Rome.
3. Ibid.
4. On this point it is strange to note that the *British Journal of Psychiatry* continues periodically to falsify the information on Trieste. See the comic article by K. Jones which is a remarkable example of incompetence and ideological distortion full of superficial statements – a revealing example of how unacceptable the Trieste results are for the British establishment. Jones, K., Poletti, A. (1986) 'The "Italian Experience" Reconsidered', *British Journal of Psychiatry*, 148, pp. 144–50.

17

Replacing Mental Hospitals with Better Services

DAVID KING

Why Mental Hospitals Must Close

The time has come to sweep away the old mental hospitals and replace them with something different and better. There are proven alternatives and the main impediment to their introduction is the time and resources lavished on forlorn efforts to reform the Victorian and Edwardian legacy of vast, isolated asylums. Everyone recognizes that these places are inappropriate, and many believe that they fail Florence Nightingale's acid test by doing more harm than good.

It is hardly surprising that they are not suitable for modern approaches to care and rehabilitation since they were built for a purpose, the lifelong containment and control of pauper lunatics – a purpose in total conflict with rehabilitation. If they had not existed they would not need to have been invented. Sadly, because they exist, they find loyal defenders of the notion that they occupy a central and crucial place in the pattern of psychiatry. There is a danger that their existence will influence any succeeding mental health systems with the idea that the best and most complex work should be done at such distant centres. This would be unfortunate for little, if anything, requires their retention. Mental health is an aspect of life where the focus should be personal and local, not distant, and where professional specialists have a contribution to make but in which they should not dominate. It will be difficult to achieve this while the mental hospitals are still in being and that is why they must go.

There is one defence of the mental hospitals which must command some respect and that is the possibility that, scattered throughout the community, those in most need of help can easily be forgotten or deliberately neglected. Sadly, too few people are aware of the impoverishment and neglect of the resident populations in the mental hospitals during the past 30 years. It appears people can be out of sight and mind either in the hospital or the community. The evidence suggests that neglect is possible whether or not the hospitals exist. However, we must insist on active and concerned mental health services which will continue to bid for what is necessary and expose attempts at official neglect.

Hospitals Can Close

For the past 125 years Exeter has been a centre of mental hospital services for the 1.5 million people of the counties of Devon and Cornwall. There are four large hospitals and about ten smaller ones, and in their prime they housed some 4,000 people. Since the mid-1950s these numbers have been falling and the hospitals have been less crowded. But as conditions improve and former residents move out it has become increasingly apparent that the hospitals have created many of the behavioural conditions they were apparently there to treat. In short, in better, more normal conditions most people respond and behave more normally. It is also apparent that much of the work undertaken centrally would be better done locally. Therefore, since 1980 it has been the health authority's policy to close down the central hospitals and distribute the services throughout the two counties.

At the time of writing (June 1986) the first large hospital, Royal Western Counties, has closed and two more are emptying for closure later this year. The idea of mental hospitals closing is not new, it has been adumbrated since the early 1960s: actual closures are still rare and there is interest both in the process and in what replaces the hospital.

What Led to the Change?

Although much fuss is made about the distinction between mental illness and mental handicap hospitals, our forebears were not aware of the difference and admitted people to either type of institution and there are remarkable similarities in the experience of managing both. In the mid 1970s the priorities for the mental hospitals in Exeter were to reduce bed complements of the crowded wards and improve the privacy and amenities for patients. Staffing levels everywhere needed improvement and the fabric of the hospitals and the service systems (heat, light and power) called for vast investment. No attempt was made to plumb this bottomless pit of demand, every penny which could be grabbed was invested to achieve the minimum standards stipulated by the DHSS. There were endless negotiations with all kinds of staff to alter their working practices to improve the patients' day. Somehow it seemed that the faster everyone bailed, the more water there was to shift.

Although there was some development of community services there was no commitment to them nor any expectation that they would relieve the intolerable pressures on the hospitals. Perhaps if any light could have been seen at the end of the tunnel, the considerable efforts to improve the hospitals would have continued, but the evidence insistently pointed to an alternative solution which at that time, if not unthinkable, was certainly unmentionable without a massive outburst of irritation and unrest: namely, to replace the hospitals with different services. But two events and a statistical trend in the late 1970s forced nearly everyone to this unpalatable conclusion.

The first was a long and detailed negotiation in only two of the large hospitals to change the shift pattern of nursing staff. A rough assessment of what remained to be done in trying to change institutional practices indicated many years of similar exhausting and expensive negotiations. The second event was a decision not simply to redecorate or 'upgrade' the wards but to remodel the two worst examples in the largest hospital. Again, this took much time and money, and the cost of making similar improvements throughout the whole hospital system would be fabulously expensive. The statistical trend showed a continuing and inexorable decline in the numbers of resident patients of all categories. It appeared that we might conceivably achieve, after great expense and enormous human effort, a perfect hospital system at about the same time as it finally emptied of all patients.

It was understood that the intended policy of the Department of Health was to have mental health and mental handicap services in every district and that they should be distributed within each district, but there were no models or extra central funding, the essential ingredients to transform policies from intentions to practice. It became clear that if things were to change in Devon and Cornwall it must be by using the resources invested in the hospitals and developing new models of service by local experiment and using whatever examples were to be found. It was not immediately clear that whole hospitals would close, only that they would scale down. The only other example of major change, the 'Worcester Experiment', had seen the introduction of considerable new resources and no reduction of existing services. However, since there was no prospect in Exeter of a major infusion of new resources, the new services throughout the five districts in Devon and Cornwall (including Exeter) could only be funded by a compensating reduction in the hospitals.

Commitment to Change

Although there had been much apparently fruitless work in Exeter in the late 1970s to improve the hospitals, it had its positive side. It was the heyday of multidisciplinary management and joint negotiation with trade unions: in consequence, a large nummber of peopple had been briefing themselves on the frustration of the hospital system and becoming aware of the likely future pattern of community-based services. Quite by accident the ground was being prepared for change. Of course, similar debates were going on in other places in the UK which did not result in a resolve to anticipate change rather than eventually be overtaken by it. The writing was on the wall for everyone to read; some chose to ignore it.

In a nutshell, the policy was that the move to more locally-based services would be made possible by the closure of the central hospitals and that everyone involved in the old system would, if they wished, have a place in the new. Three management units were set up each with new community-based services to develop and a hospital to close which would resource the change. This made a negative activity into a positive development and provided the incentives which so often are missing. The prospect of moving to the new by closing the old was so attractive that each unit set itself an ambitious timetable for change. These timetables showed simply the end-of-year targets for ward reductions and compensating community developments; six-monthly reports on progress made towards these have been presented to the health authority. The objective was clearly stated, managers appointed to do the work and a timetable established to set the pace of change and targets set for the end of each year of the projects.

However, because there was uncertainty, save in the broadest terms, about the final nature and patterns of service, the management units had considerable freedom to vary solutions and learn from both experience in Exeter and information from elsewhere. It is accepted that the first solutions are likely to be influenced too much by hospital experience and that change and adaptation must be much more a characteristic of the new services than it was of the old.

Overcoming Resistance to Change

It is possible to have all the right answers but not to be given the chance to implement them and there was concern that staff and public anxieties could well frustrate what were, for the time, quite radical plans. Fortunately, the amount of trade union involvement in work leading up to these changes meant that the ideas were not new to the local leadership; indeed they had had a major hand in formulating them. But if staff – some 2,500 in all – were to be convinced of the good sense of the proposals and that their involvement in them was more than a paper promise, then a thorough programme of briefing and a formal 'no compulsory redundancy' agreement had to be negotiated. Each management unit with local union representatives took care of its own information processes and the internal recruitment of staff to the new services. A district-wide 'no compulsory redundancy' agreement was successfully negotiated and many claim that it was this trump card which helped the union leaders to convince the majority of their members.

At any time six or more trade unions have been involved and it is great credit to them all that their joint efforts have enabled the plans to be implemented. The commitment of authority members, chief officers and other senior staff has been matched by a similar degree of commitment at all levels. Instead of presenting an endless succession of problems for higher management to solve, as in the past, problems are solved where they occur and the resourcefulness and flexibility of staff and their representative organizations is probably the most important element underpinning the success of the programmes. Two aspects in particular are worthy of comment. The first is the imaginative and flexible staffing plans the unions have been willing to negotiate, in marked contrast to previous hospital experience. The second is the comfortable and co-operative working relationships with voluntary organizations and the private sector, for with a move to the community, greater contact is inevitable, but a positive attitude to it is not necessarily guaranteed.

The public reaction to these changes suggests that efforts to create a positive response have been less successful but this may be because of the high profile given to the spasmodic alliance of critics and journalists who find in what they have to say a rich compost for controversial headlines. There has been massive public education and explanation and central to this, good understanding and support from the Community Health Council (the public's health watchdog), local elected members of parliament and councillors, and the major mental health and handicap charities.

The stumbling block is protest, which seems inevitable from neighbours whenever a household or hostel of former hospital residents is to be set up and planning permission is required. Speaking to people in the neighbourhood in advance of formal application can sometimes avert problems. Sadly, people seem to have no qualms about saying the most outrageous things of people who have been in a mental hospital, and newspapers do not hesitate to report. One outburst was so extreme that it backfired and made our task easier. There is a case for extending discriminatory legislation, if only to curb press statements. Happily, experience indicates that worries are quelled and often converted into natural goodwill after the proposed household is established.

Resources for Change

Critics of community care and those hesitant to make the change find this a most fruitful area for obstructing progress. There is the popular myth that governments expect community care to cost less, and a general assertion that it costs more. There is also the view that only with more money, and centrally-provided bridging funds, will changeover be possible. At least we can now bring factual evidence to this debate. The health authority decided at the outset to spend at least as much on the new services as it had the old. It also decided to divide the budget of the mental hospitals pro rata to the population of the districts served by the central hospitals: this meant less for Exeter than in the past, for proximity of the hospitals resulted in greater use of them by Exeter people. The relative position on the mental health budget (a service based in Exeter for three districts) works out as follows:

Table 17.1 Mental Health Budgets in Exeter (1986)

District	Before	After	% change
	£m	£m	
Torbay	2.6	4.6	+77%
N. Devon	1.3	1.8	+38%
Exeter	8.0	5.5	-31%
Total	11.9	11.9	

Exeter district benefits from a reduced share of the budget for the reasons stated above, and has set up a robust community service so that, in theory, community services will cost less in Exeter than the use it made of hospitals. Of course they are two quite different services and all that can be said is that the hospital budget has been sufficient in the three districts served to set up local services.

The inefficiencies of old hospitals have contributed to the care budget of the new-style services and modern buildings. In the service for elderly people the central hospital has been replaced by a number of small units each with beds, day places and a domiciliary team; day rates are broadly comparable between the new units and old hospitals save that overheads account for 25 per cent of costs in the former compared with 40 per cent in the latter. Small is both beautiful and, apparently, cost effective.

Of course, the real waste in terms of using money allocated for health purposes is the proportion of it spent on residential care or housing costs. Even as the hospitals are emptied, residents are still found who could, with a little support, have coped very well in the community. The case costs for a 30-year period of residence are both high and wasteful since prolonged institutionalization reduces the possibility of return to the community. Whether these changes are called 'savings' or not, it does mean there is more money available for care, which because of the greater geographical spread of service makes it accessible to more people.

Bridging funds, temporarily available to start up new services before closing the old, have been necessary. This has been managed within the district budget without any special assistance from outside agencies. The money used had been reserved to commission some new services in the general hospital and it has been released from bridging duties when the new facilities have become available. Not everyone will have this opportunity and bridging must be provided, but the solution is not insuperable – too often it seems to be used as an excuse for inactivity. The real discipline is to ensure the closure of hospital services so that funds can be transferred to the community.

Once in the community, managers quickly become expert at discovering the resources available in other sectors of the economy for housing, employment, social security grants and the like. Instead of the health budget having to fund everything as it did in hospitals, there are other resources available to the ordinary citizen.

Style of Community Services

Exeter is a city of 100,000 people surrounded by rural communities based on market towns and seaside resorts. The authority recognizes these communities and has identified 12 at present and seeks to provide each with its own broad range of services – the object is to spread into, not rationalize and withdraw from communities. Mental health and mental handicap services are ideal for this decentralized pattern of care, and community teams have been established to plan, develop and manage whatever services are required by local populations. The objective is to respond to current needs rather than manage a set of residential and day facilities to which customers must be recruited. That is the guiding principle which is by no means achieved yet.

In each locality there are public representatives (usually town or parish councillors) and customer representatives (families of mentally handicapped people, for example) who join with local professionals from health, social services and other social agencies (housing, employment) to plan and develop services. In this way it is hoped to ensure that services will remain attentive to local need and that change will be easier because everyone will have contributed to it – the services will be rooted in the community.

Many people who were behaviourally disturbed in the hospitals have settled well once returned to ordinary society and free of institutional frustrations and control, but there are others for whom this does not yet seem appropriate and facilities have been retained for this group in a district hospital unit. With this small exception the majority of services for mentally handicapped, confused elderly and mentally ill people are being provided in the localities.

The Future and Care in the Community

There is a danger in thinking that when all three hospitals are closed, the task will have been accomplished – it will not. Only a beginning has been made and the services must be regularly evaluated to avoid the stagnation experienced in the hospitals. It is now accepted that most of the other hospitals will close so that the whole of the mental handicap service will be locally-based and mental illness hospitals reduced to an essential minimum. It will be interesting to see whether it is easier to adapt and change services, particularly when mistakes have been made.

One of the most interesting challenges is providing a sympathetic service for older people – the numbers over 65 years of age exceed 20 per cent of the total population and those over 85 will continue to rise for many years yet. Increasingly, it does appear that more and more should be done to support people at home and in an ordinary life and that residential and training facilities specially provided, even at the local level, perpetuate the artificiality and unacceptability of institutional care. The constant challenge in human services is to ensure that the wishes and needs of others are given the active attention and action we would wish for our own.

18

How Can Mental Hospitals be Phased Out?

GIOVANNA DEL GIUDICE, EVARISTO PASQUALE, MARIO REALE

The psychiatric hospital in Trieste ceased to exist as such in 1980.[1] The area once taken up by it now houses a state primary school, a professional institute, a gymnasium, a bar, four university wards, music, painting and theatre laboratories and several co-operative headquarters. Three hundred and twenty long-term patients still live within this area, mainly in group homes, and they have all acquired the status of guests.

The Trieste psychiatric hospital was a model hospital. It was built in 1907, at the time of the Austro-Hungarian empire, on a hill just outside the city. The wards were tidy and bright and set within a very large park. Functional, clean and muffled like the existing hospitals in Northern Europe, it housed contradictions, suffering and shouting. It confirmed separation from the outside world which was kept at bay by gates, keys, straitjackets. It hid everything which appeared unable to be changed or retrieved for social and productive life – individuals who were socially weak.

Secrecy and obscurity had become 'the institutional order'; the workers' silence, 'capability and efficiency', the patient's silence, 'the achievement of normality'. And when the suffering quietened down and no longer burst out, access was gained to the advantages of the institution – you could go up the hill, to the high wards for 'calm patients' and 'workers', finally leaving behind the contradictions, forgotten by the world.

In 1971 there were 1,200 patients, 10 doctors, and 353 nurses. It was the nurses' job to ensure silence and order. The doctor, who was not present, regulated this work by straitjackets and drugs. Nurses referred only to the chief nurse. Order, separation, secrecy, quietening down conflicts, suffocating suffering to achieve immobility – these things kept the mental hospital alive and functioning. Closing it down, superseding it, could only mean overturning all this:

• **Life's disorder** contrasted and replaced institutional order. Relationships were no longer sustained and fixed by the mechanisms and rules of the institution. They redefined themselves as relationships with individuals who would deny and overwhelm or with those who would listen and help. These types of relationship encouraged the expression of needs and guaranteed a therapeutic relationship for each individual patient. In this way, nurses continued to control and give medicine but they also accompanied patients who felt confined by the ward, into the town and gardens and home for a few hours, for example the little old lady who, because she is far away from her usual points of reference, is in danger of senile decay in the ward.

• **Institutional openness** which exposes neglect and suffering in order to tackle them, replaced the secrecy of a world which had hidden its misery and was ashamed and afraid of it. The methods and stages of this transformation were public, visible from the 'outside'. A patient who injured him/herself after a fall in the ward was taken to the general hospital. More attention was paid to the patient's health than to the institution covering up for its workers' mistakes.

At the same time, meetings at the regional level, schools, holidays and cultural activities for the city brought the people of Trieste into the hospital. They filled the spaces and the park. They mixed with the patients who, torn from their inertia and immobility, reacquired desires, needs, the ability to relate, human faces, the desire for freedom and for their own resources.

• **Separation** from normality and from everyday life outside the hospital was overcome by introducing a great number of new professionals and very basic things – such as knives, forks, mirrors and wardrobes. These objects brought normality to a world artificially created for madness and danger.

Once the doors of the mental hospital were open, diversity and suffering were discharged into the city and required a response. This has touched and found continuity and roots in the suffering which had swamped the city. This was not only material suffering but also the absence of relationships, loneliness, the lack of health and political planning. Because these ills had been returned openly to the city, the city was able to find ways of overcoming them.

• The **conflicts** of a world no longer separate and closed burst forth in the form of inescapable needs. The illness was no longer linked to the institution but to an individual's own history which was reconstructed and which regained the right to exist. Also, the more changes to wards were introduced, the more necessary it became to guarantee recognition of the patient's needs and of workers' therapeutic capabilities, given the new uncertainty.

The conflicts burst forth in the form of institutional and cultural diffidence on the part of the former nurses. They did not know whether they could trust a power which until then had always obliged them to control and overwhelm those in their care. The critique of the psychiatric institution in Trieste was concerned with working practices and it was rooted in everyday life.

• **Everyday life** was interpreted as *attention to everyday life*. Different types of social encounters were tried which produced changes. Solidarity came about and what normally appeared incomprehensible and irretrievably broken was mended.

For these reasons, normal acts of everyday life are valued in the changing hospital more than techniques and new science which still guarantee power to the same group of professionals.

• **Everyday involvement** of all professionals in the institution's daily routine. By not delegating activities, psychiatrists in particular reassumed power through their presence which legitimized the change. In this way a patient who was agitated and refused to co-operate was managed personally without medication – even relating on a physical level, a relationship which meant recognition of the various individuals beyond the level of the mere exercise of coercion.

Rehabilitation of long-term patients took place as the layers of their institutionalization were peeled away. Patients were accompanied outside the wards to rediscover other spaces and other dimensions. The rigid separation of the sexes was broken down. And even the violent crises of the change were shared by the users. Real voices and relationships replaced the 'voices' which had previously kept patients company. Their history was reconstructed through witnesses and institutional records. They were encouraged to return to the place where they had lived before hospitalization. The city and its changes were rediscovered, as were one's own face in the mirror and one's body through one's own clothes. Spaces in the mental hospital were transformed and used in a different way. They were redecorated, furnished and filled with objects which suggested an alternative existence. Through investment in resources such as clothes, furnishings, relationships and money, the workers acquired greater professionality through the recognition of the patients' dignity and the possibility of change and cure.

Patients' capacity to relate, to express, to achieve companionship, to recognize and affirm their own rights, have emerged. This has made rehabilitation and a therapeutic relationship possible.

Because coercion was eliminated and patients were allowed to regain their civil rights, the administrative figure of the 'guest' emerged. User co-operatives were formed so that occupational therapy could be dispensed with. These co-operatives engaged in cleaning the wards and then in training new patients. The subsidy given out in the institution as charity or as an additional form of control and dependence became accepted as an 'essential minimum' for acquiring real autonomy.

The new professional status acquired by nurses during the change was ratified by economic and legal recognition. When long-term patients were discharged from the psychiatric hospital, they were accommodated in family homes which were run partly or completely by workers. The psychiatric hospital was replaced mainly by district mental health centres.

It is very important to repeat that in Trieste administrative regulations have always followed the practical changes already made. The closure of the hospital was not a bureaucratic operation but the collective effort of patients, psychiatrists, nurses and citizens who worked together on a plan to emancipate and socially regenerate individuals who had little or no social power.

For us workers, the change brought about in the mental hospital was our *main training ground*. It was here that we recognized the poverty of the psychiatry which confined social conflict and whatever had been rejected by other institutions and medical cultures. It was a stopping place on the route to marginalization, a science functioning as an instrument of social control. It denied value, significance and the right to exist of different forms of expression. Here the positive ability to 'cure' was demystified and the ability to 'take responsibility' was rediscovered. The sick existence of individuals, not illness, was recognized as the aim of psychiatry.

Today, Trieste is a city without a mental hospital. Nothing is deferred anymore. All types of suffering, ways of life, and ways of falling ill are dealt with. The response to suffering is less codified and predetermined. The roots of suffering are more easily recognized and understood as the individual's life history. Knowledge of an individual's life experiences provide a source of information which can be understood and confronted.

New principles and types of practice have developed:

The Right of Asylum
The ancient, sacred right of asylum is interpreted today as *the right to a bed* in the new district services. It has a completely different meaning from a bed in the mental hospital which was used to impose exclusion from society.

The mental health centre offers asylum to the depressed patient when s/he finds it necessary to leave the reality of home, such as the manic youth who finds the walls and relationships of home too constraining and who needs a different space which is more free and flexible; the person in acute psychotic crisis; the patient brought in by the police; and the individual in crisis with psychomotor agitation. It also accepts the need of a patient who is trying to escape the violent, competitive mechanisms of current social organization.

The Worker's and the Service's Responsibility Towards the Service User

When Law 180 was passed in 1978 it was not followed by practical regulations. Many psychiatrists who did not immediately favour the reform have tried to argue that with the closure of mental hospitals not only has custodial responsibility towards those no longer hospitalized ceased, but also therapeutic responsibility. Consequently on many occasions the professional did not take responsibility for following up constantly, and with an overall vision, a patient who had been reintroduced to the social environment. These professionals did not see their contribution as a secure alternative to internment. They did not accept the innumerable problems posed by the new 'citizens with mental illness', such as refusing care, not attending at meetings, devaluing the therapist's role and being constrained by social problems. Therefore many families and citizens who are concerned with – or feel threatened – by reintegration or non-care, protest against this irresponsibility and neglect of the users by the workers of the psychiatric services.

However, in Trieste there has been a struggle to create district structures which guarantee support round the clock for both former and new patients and their families. Inevitably this approach relies on workers who do not limit themselves to treating clinical symptoms only, but who take responsibility for all the issues which these symptoms express. Not only must they take steps to strengthen clients but also set in motion practical solutions for change.

The extreme limit of this practical responsibility concerning the user is *making therapeutic intervention compulsory*. This can happen both when the person refuses any therapeutic relationship at all – because s/he is subject to delirious illusions or to a compulsive vision of a changed world – or when s/he needs to be removed from social or institutional neglect. It is here that the real concern of a public service towards an individual can be measured. Substantial defence barriers can be put up by individuals and these have to be overcome if the service is to succeed in taking responsibility for him/her.

Law 180 does provide for compulsory health treatment but only after all efforts to persuade the person have failed. Sometimes this requires updating work which involves various social groups such as neighbours, administrators, trusted doctors and families – if an actual meeting with the person is to be achieved. In Trieste it is thought that spells of opposition in the working relationships can and should exist, so long as each person's civil rights are guaranteed. This is because such periods can act as a springboard for further development of a therapeutic relationship; a development which challenges the personal capabilities not only of the professional, but also of clerical and domestic staff.

These choices are often accompanied by the public's indifference. This indifference is a mechanism for segregation and neglect which is more violent than internment in a mental hospital. In Trieste there is also a struggle against indifference towards those on the margins of society; and towards the significance of requests for help indicated by some of the symptoms of their disorder.

Workers have to undertake the exhausting task of clashing with other institutions so that they too take responsibility for needs which they no longer pay any attention to: sometimes it is necessary to struggle to get the emergency line to respond, to get the local authority welfare services to take account of certain individuals, and to get the hospital to accept cases of physical disease in those who are mentally distressed or who are simply marginalized.

Value of the Therapeutic Community

This particular way of being part of a group is currently valued and encouraged by users of the mental health services because even on its own it has already had an amazing therapeutic effect. The workers, who themselves are used to working and thinking in groups, are aware of the great importance that revealing emotions can have on a therapeutic relationship, for example, in alleviating a crisis of anxiety or depression. They try not only to maintain a caring relationship with users but also to encourage solidarity and forms of self-help between people using the service.

Efforts are made to create an atmosphere where users listen to each other, and this atmosphere is passed on by regular users to new ones. The new patients are often fascinated to find themselves in an environment where as well as the advantages of treatment there are also those which make up the family atmosphere.

What is offered is the chance for individuals to be the prime movers in facing their illness and that of their neighbour; the chance to express or experience with others not only their symptoms but also their potential by helping each other and by co-operating with staff to manage spaces and meetings. In addition, the service tries to respond to social relationship problems – so often ignored or suppressed in the modern world – by attempting to develop the community atmosphere into more extensive sociability outside the centre.

Here, the apparent digression from the clinical can be understood if one considers the effects that the misery of human relationships and the rigid defence of an individual's own identity produce at the beginning of psychiatric pathology.

Unfortunately, the spaces created by the psychiatric service are sometimes the only places where users can sustain social relationships; and often it is not because they are incapable of socializing in 'normal' environments (which are often pathologically competitive). It is because these contacts are not catered for in the current organization of society or are difficult for the weakest individuals to establish.

Construction of the Individual Therapeutic Relationship within the Service

Although great attention is paid to community interaction, personal contact between an individual user and a single worker is also valued and encouraged. In fact the need for an individual relationship with the patient is accepted and often engineered. This need is particularly evident in the case of serious psychotic crisis and at the beginning of the individual–service interaction. It is recognized as each user's right, including the so-called 'chronic' users. The workers try to revert the condition of 'chronic' users to the acute state once more. The organization caters for a well-defined therapeutic relationship for two people by releasing a specific worker from routine work for an appropriate period.

In fact, the value placed on nurses and their transformation into therapeutic agents with new experiences and capabilities can offer a wide and varied choice for the development of individual relationships with single clients.

In this chapter, we have briefly recalled the theory and practice which enabled us to supersede the mental hospital and we have outlined the stages by which we now live in a city without a mental hospital. This stage took ten years to arrive at, a decade of innumerable difficulties, personal and collective sacrifices and achievements.

The main difficulties are echoed wherever the reform is taken seriously, as demonstrated not only in Trieste but also in Bari (see Chapter 10), Rome (see Chapter 20), Turin (referred to in Chapter 6), among the many towns in Italy which are still undergoing the transformation.[2]

The difficulties include:

- The need to convince the political, administrative, professional and civic circles that the closure of a psychiatric hospital *must* be followed simultaneously with the establishment of a neighbourhood mental health service.
- Convincing them also that these changes are not only morally an improvement, but that they also neither endanger the local population, nor create chaos or maltreatment of patients.
- The need to demonstrate that you – as a group – can actually practise what you preach by consistent and persistent action; that you do not run for cover whenever things go wrong, as they often do!
- Living for a long period with predominantly hostile politicians, professionals and public opinion, and gradually winning over some members of these groups, while yet some others become enemies.
- Convincing the scared staff and residents, or service users, by personal example that each side can indeed trust the other and has something positive to give and receive from the other.
- Not allowing one side to project the responsibility, or guilt, or blame, to another. For example, often professionals force administrators to appear to be the group which opposes the change.
- Facing and combating persistently the chronic lack of financial, manpower and residential resources. You have alternatively to beg, flatter, or threaten – or use all three tactics together – in order to get what you consider to be the bare minimum. For example, in Bari and Gravina ex-patients and staff occupied the CMHC building for some months before the relevant authority agreed to their demand to have then and there a local group home.[3]
- Living with the exhaustion and the havoc it often creates in your private life (due to the impact of mental distress and the constant need to activate a passive environment) without becoming a 'burn out' case.

We believe, and hopefully have demonstrated in this chapter, that it is possible to tackle these difficulties without being superhuman, by remembering who we are doing it for, by creating our own support systems, and by presenting and meeting new challenges.

References

1. Mauri, D. et al. (1983) *La Libertà è Terapeutica?* Feltrinelli, Milan. This book presents in full the story of the psychiatric reform in Trieste.
2 De Salvia, D., Crepet, P. (ed) (1983) *Psichiatria senza Manicomio,*

Feltrinelli, Milan. This book gives accounts of processes of change in Arezzo, Perugia, Bologna, Venice, Genoa, Portogruaro, Pordenone, Ferrara, Settimo, Taranto, Palermo and Milan.

3. Il Comitato '180' (1981) *Dossier: Piu Case, Niente Serenase: Le Lotte per la Riforma Psichiatrica in Provincia di Bari* – a compilation of newspaper cuttings of the struggle to establish group homes.

19

Mental Health Resource Centres

RICK HENNELLY

'Community' mental health centres are a relatively new form of provision in the UK but have been in operation elsewhere (the US, for example) for up to 20 years. Such centres were seen as one possible alternative to the asylum and were expected to be comprehensive in scope.

There are potential lessons to be learnt from the experience of the community mental health centre (CMHC) movement in other countries.[1] Some obvious issues are:

- The extent to which psychiatrists were employed in such settings and their adaptation to a changing role. Loss of power and status has often occurred.
- The degree of involvement of local communities in helping to manage, or participate in, centre activities.
- The difficulties involved in integrating the CMHC with pre-existing psychiatric services.
- The extent to which the CMHC was used as an institution for changing the political and social circumstances of the community in which it was located as opposed to its focus on individual 'illness'.
- The perceived lack of support given by the CMHC to the most severely disabled people using mental health services as opposed to the support provided to those less disabled.
- The insecure funding of the CMHC and the ease with which funds were cut off following their criticism as over-politicized resources which did not cater to the most needy.
- The nature of 'multidisciplinary' activity in the CMHC. Major conflicts occurred between professions struggling to achieve a power base and confusion was generated over the role of workers not belonging to a profession.

In the UK, development of the CMHC has been much more cautious and predated by a range of other services (day hospitals, day centres, hostels, group homes, community psychiatric nursing, out-patient 'treatment' etc.). Over the last few years, however, a number of facilities describing themselves as CMHCs were created. One of the best known and earliest is Brindle House in Tameside, although many others are now in operation or at the planning stage.[2] One of the major distinctions to be made between these facilities is whether they are primarily organized as a health service facility or as a social service facility. There has been no attempt yet made in the UK to provide criteria against which a service can be described or evaluated as a CMHC.[3]

Given the problems of planning, the competition of ideas, and the vexed relationship between health and local authorities and central government, the CMHC has an uncertain future. In some areas, it will be rejected as a model of service in favour of closer liaison between primary health care and district general hospital psychiatric units. In other areas where the facility is established as a health service resource, the CMHC may develop as a comprehensive and medically-integrated alternative to the asylum, preserving many of the devaluing features of traditional forms of medical intervention. Another model of mental health centre may become apparent, more likely to occur when such a facility is local authority provision. This is the 'mental health resource centre'. It will be small-scale and probably be organized around a combination of day care and residential support. It will display some of the following features:

- Explicitly non-medical responses to mental health difficulties will be promoted.
- The experiences of power and powerlessness will be recognized as the central elements around which the theory and practice of mental health care is constructed.
- There will be an active policy of encouraging dialogue, negotiation and information flows between individuals, groups and agencies forming the mental health support network.
- Flexibility will be the keystone of organization, with individually tailored responses sought to individually experienced crisis. The search for technocratic or prescribed solutions to 'category disorders' (schizophrenia, depression, etc.) will be relegated in favour of an understanding of unique experiences.
- There will be a policy of promoting the organization and strength of the 'survivors' movement (where 'survivors' refers to those people

who have managed to 'survive' life crisis and psychiatric intervention). Self-advocacy could be a related core principle of service delivery.

- Intervention will aim at 'short-circuiting' medical cycles of control, i.e. intervention will take place at the primary health and out-patients levels of activity with the aim of preventing people embarking on psychiatric 'careers'.

In the next section a centre will be described which reflects a concern with some of the above issues. Earlier descriptions of the service and the tensions between ideology and practice are contained in papers presented to the National MIND Annual Conferences 1984 and 1985.[4]

The Mental Health Services Project, Tontine Road, Chesterfield

The project employs the equivalent of five full-time social workers, part-time clerical and cleaning staff, and a varying number of part-time 'flexible care' workers. Significant features of the project include:

- Access to 'flexible care' support. Project workers, in conjunction with social services area office staff, help plan for the needs of people disabled by virtue of mental health problems. Assessment of individual need is undertaken and people specifically employed to work flexibly with the identified individuals in order that the need is met in as 'normal' an environment as possible. This facility can be used to prevent institutionalization or to help reintegration after a period of institutional living.
- Liaison with the four community mental health teams which together respond to 'acute' breakdowns in a 280,000 catchment population area across North Derbyshire.
- A commitment by project workers to help establish and support social support networks across the North Derbyshire Health District.
- The existence of a set of service principles based upon the results of research into the needs of people using mental health services prior to the introduction of the project, as well as the Derbyshire County Council Social Services Department policy of promoting ordinary life for ex-patients. The work of the project is influenced by the guidelines for normalization work proposed by O'Brien.[5]

It is worth noting that most of the people who experience crises of mental health do not live in hospitals. Networks of support organized around and with such individuals promise the opportunity of creating extended groups of people who are educated about the social and political aspects of medical care, psychotropic drug use, hospitalization, and the value of ordinary human support in times of crisis. This information will help these individuals, and others whom they in turn influence, negotiate the circuits of medical control experienced at primary health, out-patient and in-patient levels of 'psychiatric care'.

As indicated already, power and powerlessness are central elements around which theory and practice may be constructed. People who have mental health crises most commonly experience a sense of powerlessness and loss of control. The experience of being medically treated is singularly inappropriate under these circumstances since such treatment often reinforces such experiences. In order to improve the service we offer to people, it may be helpful to analyse our actual encounters with people who come to us seeking support, as well as more general features of mental health services, in terms of the exercise of power in key areas where the interests of different groups are represented.

Our Own Power and How We Deal with it
Our own power is experienced in a variety of ways: we handle resources such as a development budget which is used to financially support groups in the district with a mental health interest; we are invested with power by people who come to the service seeking help; we experience power in our everyday involvements with people using our services, such as the avoidance of eye contact by someone who perceives paid workers as frightening and powerful.

In an environment geared to the exploration of emotional events and a culture of mutual support where, as workers, we 'own up' to ordinary experiences and the inadequacy of 'professionalism', we are sometimes asked how we maintain an 'appropriate' emotional distance. For instance, can there be legitimacy in an intimate relationship between a 'worker' and a 'client' or is the worker inevitably abusing his/her position of power? This is the question put from the standpoint of professional ethics. Social workers, clerical staff, students, voluntary sector workers using the building, flexible care workers who use the resource on an occasional basis, people who are very dependent, people who define themselves as having overcome their personal stresses, people who define themselves as 'volunteers' (even though the term is discouraged), are all part of the centre. They become part of an increasingly complex picture of activity where change is the order of things and 'worker/client' distinctions, as traditionally conceived, are not easily made. The question then becomes a different one: is it possible to have some guidelines or principles by which a network of individuals, who have very different experiences of power and responsibility, can make judgements about the behaviour of individuals within that network related to close emotional ties?

How We Attempt to Empower People Using Services

One way to do this is to collectively empower people using services. This means giving groups a set of choices over their own activities and the deployment of resources. For instance, organizing a major social event is a complicated activity requiring many different decisions to be made and allowing for the involvement of many people taking different levels of responsibility.

Historically the paid workers of the Mental Health Services Project were associated with the support of a fairly large group of people using the Tontine Road Centre for a variety of social, educational, recreational and occupational activities. As the group grew in confidence and developed a more formal structure (rites of entry, community meetings etc.) we conceived the idea of 'normalizing' relations between the project and the people using the service.

After discussions, some major changes occurred during the first half of 1985. The group now has a name, CONTACT, and a formal, written constitution. The constitution allows for elections to an executive committee comprising four men and four women. Ultimate authority rests with the weekly organized community meeting. Along with these changes, after negotiation with the workers of the project, nearly £2,000 was given to the group to enable it to organize its own activities. This is a small first step but a significant one.

This situation has many advantages. The group now has the same formal status as the other voluntary sector groups, and can book rooms and use the premises without the 'need' for paid workers to be present all the time. The concept of 'membership' of a well-defined group has less stigmatizing connotations than does 'patient' or 'client' status. Written rules for the group make the boundaries of acceptable behaviour clear to newcomers and give a clear mandate for the 'leaders' of the group to take action if individuals offend the group. The only formal control the group has over its own members is exclusion.

The formal assumption of responsibility by the group for its own activity has allowed project workers to become more involved in developing similar networks of support. In the outlying districts we have been able to provide advice with formal organizational development and the provision of financial grants to enable similarly empowered groups to come into being. These developments allow for the provision of locally delivered services. Although this form of organization makes our role as workers a more marginal one, we do not envisage as yet the complete withdrawal of our involvement from these groups. Sensitive and complex issues regularly arise within these networks requiring protracted negotiation and dialogue between members where we are called upon to play a part in exploring the power relations involved and the balancing of 'rights'. We are thus in a transitional stage where a comprehensively organized group controlled by survivors is still aimed at rather than achieved.

Expulsion of group members is one of the issues where we are called upon to 'arbitrate'. Paid workers may have knowledge of resources over and above those commanded by the group considering expulsion, and may be able to suggest solutions which do not involve the complete withdrawal of support from those people who have consistently 'crashed' the boundaries set by the group.

Another issue requiring participation by paid workers at times is the promotion of discussion concerned with the identification of the specific needs of women and of disadvantaged minorities. Their interests need to be assertively stated and a link can then be made between the experience of powerlessness in the context of being 'treated' by the mental health services and in the context of membership of a disadvantaged group.

How We Attempt to Empower the Community

'Community' here simply means the population of a geographical area. Empowering communities entails the involvement of many community members and activists in the identification of need, and building on the abilities and strengths inherent in the community towards the meeting of these needs. It also involves community members in gaining control over the resources available to meet need.

We have taken part in a variety of activities which relate in some way to this issue. Supporting the development of voluntary sector groups and recognizing their importance is one method. In Chesterfield, our involvement with groups such as the local branch of the National Schizophrenia Fellowship and Care for Carers (for carers of elderly people with mental health problems) has been fairly substantial. These are two of the 32 voluntary groups using the community centre. Access to meeting rooms, printing facilities and financial help are the more obvious forms of support. The dangers of such close involvement by statutory workers in the voluntary sector have been well documented and will not be detailed here. Therefore we focus on providing information to these groups about their rights and about the way in which they can influence the attitudes of health and social services workers and the types of services provided.

A more recent development in democratizing and extending dialogue about the planning of services has been the formation of mental health local planning groups. Each of these groups serves a population with an average of 70,000 people (still too large for our liking) to cover the four sectors comprising North Derbyshire. These groups consist of a wide variety of statutory workers (community mental health teams, social workers from area offices, probation, education and housing representatives, GPs, mental health services project workers and so on) and representatives of groups using services. The terms of reference are loosely defined but request local planning groups to help assess local need and to feed back their findings to managerial joint planning mechanisms.

Commonly a debate about how local need should be assessed has begun and different methods of tackling the problem tried out. One sector has amassed a wide range of statistical information which give clues to local need. Another is attempting to construct a questionnaire which will be widely distributed. In both instances attempts were also made to identify and list those resources which already existed.

Strengths already exist in local communities in a variety of forms. Building on these without overburdening them or 'colonizing' natural support systems is of key importance in community mental health work. Our project has its own budget which is used to give financial aid to relevant community organizations, and Derbyshire County Council sets aside an annual 'Community Self-Help Fund' which is also used to provide initial funding for community concerns. The printshop at the project provides cheap printing facilities to community groups.

How We Relate to the Power of Management

Key problems for grassroots workers in welfare agencies which attempt to introduce innovative practice are the power and attitudes of management. Refusal to take risks, demands for operational accountability, financial restrictions and general institutional demands of the departments in which practitioners work, can all prevent change and the implementation of radical ideas.

We have found ourselves in the fortunate position of being a project which has been empowered to a degree which is unusual within a state social services department setting. This has come about for many reasons: the historical inadequacy of mental health provision in North Derbyshire before 1981 required rapid remedial measures; the background of the project co-ordinator as an influential advocate of the rights of social services employees; the ideological commitment of the workers to autonomy and democratic self-management; the political pressure, created by 'care in the community' policies on the social services department to demonstrate its commitment to service provision and need for a strong profile in relation to health authority developments. The possibilities which were opened up by the determination of newly elected representatives to save and extend services in county council elections in 1981 have contributed too.

The 'normal life' strategy adopted by the county authorities was financially backed up by a 'flexible care' budget. This made available sums of money to be used to appoint people to work with named individuals in the community who needed support at any time of the day due to being at risk of hospitalization. A great deal of discretion was given to project workers in the construction of 'flexible care' planning and appointment of suitable personnel. This in turn laid the basis for a policy of building on natural networks of support. Money was also made available on an annual basis for project staff to use at their discretion to support the development of groups in the community providing mental health services.

The social services management also agreed to the formation of the group of people using the service as an independently constituted body and accepted that such a body had a right to control its own finances.

Having said this, it must be pointed out that there are problems. Any new service responding to need in a new way causes contradictions for a pre-existing welfare bureaucracy. For example, we have an ideological commitment to maximizing the amount of social contact with groups of people using services which has led us to cut down our time spent on record-keeping and administrative tasks. In turn, this implies a minimal use of office space and an 'open door' policy in relation to use of the available office space. This places great demands on administrative workers, who have become key personnel in delivering services. Such responsibilities are not recognized by a management which has no framework for rewarding the central involvement of this group of people. This has resulted in a prolonged struggle to have their departmental status revised.

How We Cope With the Power of Other Services

GPs, generic social workers, community mental health team members and ward-based nursing staff also provide mental health services on behalf of the state. Given this diversity, conflicts arise and power struggles are played out. Co-ordination of activity and ease of communication with other agencies are large problems for specialist mental health facilities. Almost inevitably, for ourselves the greatest tension appears to arise with medical-somatic service. The slow death of the asylum is rendering the ideological conflict between the 'medical model' and a 'sociopolitical' model of mental health distress more apparent and more widespread.

Practitioners who emphasize social factors as influences on well-being, who argue the right for all of us to be able to make choices in our health care, who stress the need to extend democratic decision-making about service provision, and who are committed to removing the myths surrounding the activity of 'professionals as technicians', open the door to criticism from those who wish to cling to powerful positions. How do we cope with the dangers of being personally and collectively isolated and victimized?

- We can provide solutions to problems which involve group exploration using dialogue and negotiation.
- We can change our relationships towards people turning to us or our service by building on their strengths and abilities and building on our shared experiences with these people.
- We can support the emergence of participation by 'recipients' of mental health services and relevant charitable and institutional groups such as MIND, National Schizophrenia Fellowship, the Church organizations.
- We can refuse to collude in activities which exclude people who use services and which seek to create 'classes' within our services.
- We can continually seek to build alliances with groups of people who use services and who show an inclination towards self-organization. We can let them use facilities we have access to, or help them get their own.
- Essentially and centrally, we can establish a network of individuals, or join an established network, with whom we can share anxieties, successes, frustrations, problems, solutions etc.
- We can spread information about good 'alternative' practices in mental health.
- We can use a language which omits references to discriminatory attitudes and values or unhelpful and devaluing labels such as 'chronic schizophrenic'.
- We must recognize the social and political dimensions of our work and act upon them, by using trade union organizations, by forming contacts with sympathetic councillors elected to health and social services committees, by arguing for our employer to have a set of principles by which services are delivered.

- We can strive to effect change *with*, not *to*, people who use mental health services, and need to recognize that the struggle to transform and defend the health and social services is the same struggle to transform and improve the existence of those whose lives are affected by the operation of these institutions.

There are still difficulties to be faced. When people are trying to use different models flexibly and display their confusion about these conflicting models in ways which are unacceptable to authoritarian practitioners, they are often described as 'manipulative' and may be rejected or punished. Counselling on the value or otherwise of the major tranquillizers is another major area of contention.

Conclusion

'Mental health resource centres' are likely to be a new form of response to the changing demands of mental health service delivery. They will differ from the concept of 'community mental health centre', as that term is usually understood, on the basis of certain characteristics; they will not aim at comprehensiveness, they may not be multidisciplinary, and their ideology is likely to be sociopolitical. They are not simply reducible to day centres as they will differ in certain crucial respects; the boundaries to involvement will be much more fluid, there will be a significant outreach component, some form of residential support may be built in, the educational component will be greater, and there will be more active involvement from members of local communities.

Finally, for 'community mental health' to have real meaning, issues about the distribution of power in our services must be addressed, as I have attempted to do above. Whether we are obliged to receive services or whether we are paid to deliver them, our sense of control, confidence and ability to act constructively is crucially influenced by our perception of our own power and the boundaries to the power of others. To the extent that we can influence the institutional forces which constrain our action, we will feel a sense of belonging, and a sense of allegiance, to the service of which we are a part.

References

1. For instance, see:
    Beigel, A. (1982) 'Community Mental Health Centers: A Look Ahead', *Hospital and Community Psychiatry*, vol. 33, no. 9, September.
    Borus, J. (1978) 'Issues Critical to the Survival of Community Mental Health', *American Journal of Psychiatry*, 135:9, September.

Brown, P. (1985) Chapter 3, *The Neotraditional Public Sector: Community Mental Health Centers in The transfer of Care*, Routledge & Kegan Paul, London.

Dowell, D., Ciarlo, J. (1983) 'Overview of the Community Mental Health Centers Program from an Evaluation Perspective', *Community Mental Health Journal*, vol. 19, no. 2, summer.

Fagin, L. (1985) 'Deinstitutionalization in the USA', *Bulletin of the Royal College of Psychiatrists*, vol. 9, June.

Feldman, S. (1978) 'Promises, Promises or Community Mental Health Services and Training: Ships that pass in the night', *Community Mental Health Journal*, vol. 14, no. 2, summer.

Mollica, R. (1980) 'Community Mental Health Centres: an American response to Kathleen Jones', *Journal of the Royal Society of Medicine*, vol. 73, December, pp. 863–70.

Pardes, M., Stockdill, J. (1984) 'Survival Strategies for Community Mental Health Services in the 1980s', *Hospital and Community Psychiatry*, vol. 35, no. 2, February, pp. 127–32.

Rumer, R. (1978) 'Community Mental Health Centres: Politics and Therapy,' *Journal of Health Politics*, Policy and Law, vol. 2, no. 4, winter.

2 McAusland, T. (ed) (1985) 'Planning and Monitoring Community Mental Health Centres', King's Fund, February.

3. King's Fund Centre (1985) Background papers for Community Mental Health Centres and Community Mental Health Teams – *Tackling the Key Issues*, Workshop, December.

4. Milroy, A., Hennelly, R., Background papers to MIND annual conference (1984), 'Exploiting Infinity' and (1985) 'Changing our Ways', Mental Health Services Project, Chesterfield.

5. O'Brien, J. (1983) *Community Support Systems for People with Severe Mental Disabilities*, background paper for the King's Fund Workshop: Planning Local Psychiatric Services, September.

20

Community Mental Health Services in Rome

TOMMASO LOSAVIO

Up until 1978 Rome had offered two apparently separated services for mental health problems. It was easy to distinguish between the public and the private sector; the latter had been particularly developed after the Second World War and especially during the economic boom of the 1960s. On the one hand there was a public mental hospital with almost 2,000 patients, a private mental hospital but run by a religious order with another 1,000 patients, and a hospital for 'the chronic but calm insane' which was administrated by the province of Rome. However, periodically, shortage of beds meant that the psychiatric hospital was transferring groups of patients to other hospitals outside the city, on the basis of arbitrary criteria drawn up by the health authority.

The private service (with about 1,500 beds) on the other hand consisted of 'neuropsychiatric' nursing homes – some luxurious and unsubsidized, others less luxurious and subsidised by middle class health insurance schemes only (for example, those for public sector employees, journalists, executives in quasi-public sector organizations) and finally others which were in fact often neglected and poor like the public mental hospitals and subsidized by manual workers' health insurance schemes.

There was also the university, where the psychiatric clinic was located. It consisted of two wards with about 40 beds for patients, carefully selected according to the field of research currently in fashion, and an admission ward which carried out a filtering function by allocating patients to the psychiatric hospital, the private nursing homes and the university wards.

There was also a district structure – one only for the whole city and the province – in the form of the mental hygiene centre which, with an extremely limited number of workers, monitored discharged patients who had been the subjects of 'experiments' in the psychiatric hospital. Finally, there was a complicated network of private specialist clinics which were dependent on the public hospitals and the university.

As already mentioned, the two services were only apparently separate because in fact the majority of nursing homes, subsidized or not, belonged to or were managed by the directors and consultants in the public psychiatric hospitals and the university. This large group of psychiatrists was fascinated by the cultural model of German psychiatry prevalent before the Second World War and the great majority of them were inclined towards a strictly biological model of mental distress. This followed the Italian tradition too; the first experiments with ECT were made in Rome in the 1940s. These psychiatrists were not very interested in the changing psychiatric treatment which was then conducted in other Italian cities, preferring not to be involved in it at all.

Thus, until the introduction of the reform in 1978, psychiatric treatment in Rome was based almost exclusively upon:

- Hospitalization (in public or private settings)
- Treatment, principally of a biological nature (ECT and drugs)
- The absence of any sort of social welfare
- The absence of any practice and culture of intervention outside
- Total institution.

It is for these reasons that the change brought about by the new law posed much more complex and dramatic problems for Rome than for other parts of Italy.

Since hospitalization became a rare option because of the new regulations, and as no other provision existed, some very serious situations arose for clients, their families and for the workers in the psychiatric services. These were workers who mostly had chosen to work in the first district services which had been hastily and arbitrarily organized by the local administration in order to comply with the regulations of the new law.

Out-patient clinics with an insufficient number of ill-prepared workers were hastily set up and arbitrarily located and were open to the public for only a few hours a day. The available three psychiatric services for voluntary and compulsory admissions were not adequate for the urgent admissions – located in the general hospital – which had been previously dealt with by the psychiatric hospitals. They could not maintain the minimum of credibility necessary for a new cultural model of psychiatric work in competition with the old model. Even though the old model had been criticized and opposed, it had had deep roots in a well-established culture, practice and economy.

This period of transition in Rome coincided with a very critical stage in the radical change of the whole structure of health care, when in 1980 local health units (USL) were created, as a result of the introduction of the Italian NHS. The metropolitan district was divided into 20 such relatively autonomous units for the planning and administration of health services in a district, with each consisting of 150,000 inhabitants on average. The provincial administration which until then had administered the public psychiatric service consigned to each USL the small number of fragile structures in the psychiatric field which it had managed to set up in the previous year.

From then on Rome also was able to start a psychiatric service aimed at the district level which was at least homogeneous from an administrative point of view, if not from social, cultural and economic perspectives.[1] In each local unit the mental health departmental services (as they were now called) initiated cultural and welfare measures, often based on very diverse structures.

The diversity did not always relate to the different characteristics of the work context. Instead it was linked to former experience, to the cultural roots of the workers. Further, it depended on the degree of sensitivity of each USL administrator and on the determination of the service manager to create new solutions, to search for new structures and to establish new services. At times this implied a considerable increase in workload and relied on workers' willingness.

All this took place without a national or regional health plan and without efficient or effective co-ordination on the part of the Rome local authority which was governed by the political Left until 1985.

At the same time as the various mental health services were trying to structure themselves and achieve credibility, spontaneous bodies were growing up in the city – some supporting the Reform, others involved in investigating its contents (especially those which were more innovative). One of these innovations came into being with the establishment of the Committee for the Application of Law 180 in Rome. Members consisted of representatives of *Psichiatria Democratica, Magistratura Democratica*, the Communist Party, the Radical Party, *Democrazia Proletaria*, the Italian General Confederation of Workers (or CGIL, a Left-wing union) and relatives' associations, senior citizens, Catholic and workers' associations.

Also in Rome two major relatives' associations (DIAPSIGRA and ARAP) were created. They opposed the new law and managed to stir up affiliations in Rome and in other Italian cities. The deficiencies which they were condemning arose mainly from the potential neglect which the relatives might suffer without the psychiatric hospitals. In fact, the new services did not offer very much by way of reassurance to relatives, especially as they consisted mainly or exclusively of out-patient clinics. Above all they did not offer the sanctuary that had been guaranteed by the psychiatric hospital.

Matters were made even more difficult by the fact that only three psychiatric units were opened in three general hospitals in the city. Each service was unable to provide more than 15 beds; it meant that only 45 beds were available for more than 1,500,000 inhabitants.[2] For a variety of reasons, such as poor administration, the interests of private nursing homes, cultural resistance to admitting mental patients in general hospitals, an inadequate service was provided for those who were admitted in an acute phase for either voluntary or compulsory treatment. However, in this complex and difficult situation some teams succeeded in organizing themselves in a better way and set up in their districts an overall structure of services aimed at prevention, treatment and rehabilitation in the mental health field.

Two services aimed at crisis intervention were opened outside the hospital structures; mental health centres began to filter users to subsidized nursing homes, and attempted to monitor their own patients during the hospitalization period. Three day centres for therapy and rehabilitation were opened; most district services began to be open throughout the day and night; rehabilitation services were developed both for those still in the psychiatric hospital in preparation for their discharge and for people with a long-term disability in the district. The first preventive services were created by working within other district structures, such as the schools, parishes and workplaces, or alongside other health workers such as GPs, and those in infant and child development services, women's clinics and rehabilitation centres for people with physical handicaps.

The new services gradually acquired credibility thanks to the growing professional expertise of the workers. The latter are a mixture of older workers from psychiatric hospitals and younger ones, especially psychologists. In addition, a new model for psychiatric treatment is being developed which will supersede the traditional models (biological-psychological-social). The new model tries to respond in an overall way to mental distress by involving the client's family, his/her environment and other health and social services as well as the person him/herself.

The regional body for epidemiological research started monitoring the activities of all 20 mental health departmental services in 1984. In the same period some research was begun by the National Research Council (CNR) into the modes of functioning of these services, the types of requests made and the responses provided, and new processes of chronicity.[3]

In 1985 the Lazio region (of which Rome is a part) finally passed a law in line with many other Italian regions which outlines in precise terms the new type of district services, the way in which they are regulated, the time scale and mechanisms for closing public and private hospitals, as well as the private nursing homes. It also provides specific funding and formulates staff allocations according to the geographic and demographic characteristics of the area.

It would appear that finally, after seven years, we are coming out of a period of ad hoc solutions and confusion and that it is now possible to plan and create new services within a precise legal framework.

To illustrate, a brief description of one of the 20 mental health departments in Rome, in the 19th USL of Rome, is given below.[4] This district is located north west of the city and according to a 1981 census 185,000 people live there. It is divided into several manual worker/proletarian districts (Ottavia-Primavalle), some lower middle-class districts and into newly urbanized areas. In 1980 there was only one mental health out-patients' clinic which was only open a few days a week and for only a few hours a day. Currently, the departmental service is made up of:

- Two mental health centres open 12 hours during weekdays continuously (8am-8pm) and 6 hours a day on Saturdays and Sundays (8am-2pm). There are about 25 workers in each centre (doctors, nurses, psychologists and social workers);
- A day centre for people in an acute crisis. This centre is open for up to 12 hours during holiday periods. It is run by four psychologists and four nurses. The ratio of staff to patients is two to one, enabling the high level of attention which is required.

M., a young woman, has been brought in by her father and brother, screaming that she was being murdered by them. While one worker talked to the relatives, two others attempted to calm M. It was then proposed to her that she could stay in the centre for a few days without her relatives, to enable everyone to understand better what had happened. In the next few days M. was given medication, talked incessantly to the workers but refused to see her relatives. She cried and screamed alternately, but did not attempt to hurt herself or others. In the evening she would go to the home of a distant relative, towards whom she did not express negative feelings. After a week she was able to join in the group activities which are on offer at the centre. After two more weeks she went back home, and we started to meet with her and her family on a regular basis.

- One unit at the general hospital with 15 beds for crisis admission and for people undergoing voluntary or compulsory treatment.
- Three group homes which receive up to 12 people who have been discharged from hospitals;
- One lodging house where 35 elderly ex-patients are living;
- Two rehabilitation departments in the old psychiatric hospital where 45 ex-patients who have been discharged from the psychiatric hospital are currently waiting to be integrated into the district and use the old wards as a hostel. The wards have been turned into individual rooms. For the first time in his life, R., who was born in the hospital, had a room to himself. He decorated it with the help of other residents and staff, and was very pleased with the result. R. is working now outside the hospital with a group of residents who are responsible for gardening work in the area's public parks.
- An experiment in work rehabilitation for ex-patients, run as a therapeutic community. It is partly funded by the EEC social fund.

All of these structures, the activities taking place in them and the work of all the workers (100 in all) are co-ordinated on a departmental basis and the aim is to identify common objectives and to provide common working methods. The various professionals work on a team basis which aims to maximize the value of each worker and provide an overall response from the service. Each year about 350 new referrals (including self-referrals) are received by the service with a rise in requests from districts which have traditionally used the private sector. The service also administers summer holidays for groups of service users, distributes financial benefits and promotes cultural activities on a joint basis with a local cultural association.

In-service training and refresher courses are based on frequent team meetings where clinical, organizational and planning topics are discussed, and on the contribution of a few external supervisors. In addition, an agreement has been reached with a medical school for specialization in psychiatry aimed at training those specializing within the mental health district service structures.

The creation of this comprehensive service was focused on three objectives: replacing the psychiatric hospital and other forms of institutionalization; minimizing as much as possible the control aspect without delegating the responsibility to yet another service; avoiding as much as possible the risk of abandoning users.

We need to ask how and why it was possible to establish such a comprehensive framework in a relatively short time since 1980, on the background of the difficult situation prevailing in Rome. The question becomes particularly poignant as no other district of Rome has managed to do so on the same scale, some due to lack of desire for such a service.

There is no short and simple answer to this question. In part, it is due to the determination and professionalism of the staff group. In part it is the result of skilful work at the political-administrative level, where most of the difficulties seem to lie. In part it was the outcome of having a shared vision by a team which has undertaken the role of the protagonist in the attempt to activate every possible internal and external resource.

Considerable effort has been put into securing the movement of workers from one sector of the service to another, ensuring that at the end of the process most workers will have an insider's global perspective of the service, its users and workers. Equally we focused on the institutional and political role of the worker, his/her internal relationships and the ability to have a comprehensive perspective of the problems related to a state of suffering.

The active use of external resources was a consequence of using all of what there was: determination, obstinacy, continuous attempt to confront those in political-administrative power in order to open up new possibilities. Obviously all of this calls for an enormous personal and collective investment, resulting in creating the possibility to change what has been hitherto unchangeable, to transform not only the service but also the 'illness', to involve and to remain involved, to heal but also to 'heal oneself'.

References

1. Crepet, P., Losavio, T., Piccione, R. (1981) 'Community Mental Health Services in Rome. General Approach', ecc. in *Methodology in Psychotherapy Research*, Von Wolf H., Minsel, R., Lonhman, J. Trier, vol. 1.

2. Losavio, T. (1986) 'Il servizio psichiatrico in ospedale generale', *Lavoro Neuropsichiatrico*. Nuova Serie 1.

3. Piccione, R., Losavio, T. (1975) 'Cronicità o Lungodegenza', *Rivista Psichiatrica* X, 5.

4. Servizio Salute Mentale USL Roma 18 and 10 (1981) *Servizio di urgenza: una esperienza territoriale di superamento dei servizi di diagnosi e cura ospedalieri, Su la crisi in psichiatria,* ed Provincia di Milano.

21

Developing an Alternative Community Mental Health Service

MIND MANCHESTER GROUP

In this chapter, we concentrate on the issues that face workers in today's mental health services. There is a broad consensus amongst government bodies, professional organizations and pressure groups, that some of the resources currently committed to hospital services for the mentally ill should be transferred into the community. How exactly this is to be carried out and what it will mean for workers is not yet clear. There are important clues, however, which lead us to believe that there is a grave danger that the development of a community care system, as currently envisaged, will in reality differ little from today's hospital-based system. Except perhaps for isolated examples of good practice and the closure of the more unacceptable institutions, there is unlikely to be any radical shift in direction or philosophy.

For those people (including the authors) who are committed to the development of a community mental health service, this is profoundly depressing, but it is important we recognize these realities before we can challenge current developments in a meaningful way. We believe it *is* possible to create the foundations of a mental health service based on the principle of human dignity and the right to personal autonomy. The success of this challenge depends to a large part on the willingness of workers to examine their current and future roles. The debate about the role of workers is essentially a political one, and it would be a falsehood to portray these issues as being entirely professional. So far it has been in the interests of both 'professionals' and 'the public' to collude in confining mental health within the arena of neutral professionalism. We believe accepting the political nature of the debate leads to a direct challenge to the current organization and treatment practices of 'psychiatric services' and also a challenge to our social, economic and political life.

For those people who are sceptical about the likelihood of the success of such a challenge we would point to the experience of *Psichiatria*

Democratica in Italy, described by the Italian contributors to this book. This organization of progressive mental health workers launched a wide ranging political campaign committee to bring about change from the bottom up, i.e. involving ordinary people. For them the closure of hospitals is not just a professional issue, it is also a political and moral one.

Most workers (and the majority are not psychiatrists within 'psychiatric services') have no control over the changes taking place. They have not played an important part in determining what kind of service should replace the predominantly hospital-based system we have today. This is a reflection of the way the health service is organized with low priority placed on worker (and even less on consumer) participation in determining policy. This is a major barrier to meaningful change, particularly for those workers trying to change the existing system. As a psychiatric nurse from Manchester told us recently:

> For psychiatric nurses, ancillary workers and users, the planning and consultation machinery is irrelevant and mystifying. Most people know little or nothing about proposed changes except through their trade unions, and then often at a stage when it is too late to act constructively. We have little or no stake in the decision-making processes at all.

These dilemmas are part of an overall problem that affects today's health service. As Jim Read said in an article published in January 1985 in *Social Work Today*:

> Today's mental health service is dominated by a medically trained elite of consultant psychiatrists and run by staff whose training best equips them for operating an official hospital regime, with priority given to bed-making rather than empathy and emotions.[1]

The health service is characterized by the competing needs of the various 'professional' and 'non-professional' bodies working within it. Administrators, ancillary staff, nurses, doctors and social workers are organized within separate unions and professional associations. There is often conflict between groups of workers, particularly over changes in the service that may alter status or conditions of work. Trade unionists find themselves continually forced into reactive stances to defend jobs and existing services and in the subsequent atmosphere of mistrust, changes are opposed by workers that might otherwise be supported. The result is a service that lacks coherence, suffers from disunity and is largely undemocratic.

The challenge to progressive workers within such a system (who want to promote non-hospital alternatives) must appear to be overwhelming and even more so for those people using the service. Meanwhile, the Conservative government is busy dismantling the NHS through a process of resource starvation and privatization. This same government is also promoting community care and hospital closure, but no adequate funding has been made available to ensure that it can be accomplished. This has led to the understandable fear that by promoting community care initiatives, there is a real danger of colluding with the government's efforts to undermine the health service. The consequent difficulties of working within a neglected service with insufficient resources to do a decent job, and within depressing and inappropriate environments, has led to low morale and despondency. Hardly surprising then, that many committed workers have left the service in disgust or just 'do the job' and divorce their politics from the workplace. The centrally inspired plans for hospital closure and replacement through community care initiatives are at best regarded with scepticism, and at worst, with outright hostility.

These are not good starting points for developing a community mental health service! The factors we have described above obviously work against a creative examination of the roles of workers (or anyone else) – so where is a good starting point? As we have said, the challenge to workers is not only a professional one, it is a challenge to basic assumptions about the role mental health services play in our society.

The influence of the 'psychiatric system' affects all of us, extending far beyond the 200,000 people admitted into psychiatric hospitals each year or the millions more prescribed mind-altering drugs. Mental illness is regarded as a problem of the individual and most forms of treatment serve to isolate and stigmatize those people regarded as mentally ill. Small wonder, then, that most of us are extremely wary about discussing our own mental health openly. We are inhibited not only by ignorance and fear but also by a 'medicalized' mental health service which sees people almost exclusively as patients. Workers within this service cope only by depersonalizing the people they are there to help by labelling them according to their diagnosed illness. It is our view that current psychiatric services are doing little to counter these issues and in fact are perpetuating them through inaction and inappropriate action.

The psychiatric services themselves (as well as mental illness) invoke fear in people which prevents us from being open about our experiences. For example, ex-patients can be frightened of losing their jobs if their employers were to know they had been hospitalized. Families and friends of patients who have been made to feel powerless to help end up feeling inadequate and guilty, and usually silent. On a wider level many of us fear hospital as a consequence of others' experiences which can prevent us from taking risks or escaping from personally damaging experiences. Psychiatric services have medicalized ordinary human experiences like anger, crying, being different, idealistic, stepping out of line, and if the experiences are regarded as excessive they can result in hospitalization. Whilst withdrawal, depression, confusion and anxiety and other forms of distress do overwhelm us and become personally destructive, any help we need must be balanced against the fact that these are genuine reactions to things that go wrong in our lives.

For too long we have been socially conditioned to suppress our real feelings; it would seem that to be normal requires us to be wary about sharing our anxieties and guilts. We are being asked to believe by society (and the message is reinforced by the psychiatric services) that emotional well-being is *only* a personal issue. We emphatically deny this: for us mental health is both personal and political. It is no coincidence that the groups of people most oppressed within our society are so highly represented as users of the mental health system. What the 'psychiatric services' currently offer – the drugs, the sections and the therapies – are among the main reasons why we do not share our private anxieties and as Jim Read puts it:

> Capitalism depends too much on turning love and happiness into rare commodities. The change we want, the wresting back of control over our own lives, will come more readily if everyone recognizes the part the mental health system plays in keeping us all in our place and we challenge it at every opportunity.[2]

The first challenge to workers is to recognize that today's 'psychiatric service' is part of the problem, not the solution. It is extremely unlikely that the health service as an institution will identify these issues as significant or set goals to resolve them. Development will only occur through the organization of workers who seek change in alliance with other groups in society, developing their own agendas for action and adopting strategies to bring about a re-examination of mental health as a social and political issue. We are not naive about the enormity of this task. But we believe that only if the political implications of the mental health service are recognized, can a firm base be established on which progressive workers can build up a campaign for change.

Development of a community mental health service in this mould would inevitably meet a lot of resistance from workers within the existing 'psychiatric health service'. The current attitudes and skills of workers are best fitted to the system we have and many workers have too much investment in the existing service to welcome change; others because of poor working conditions get little job satisfaction and are apathetic and disinterested.

There will be a need to negotiate with workers that a change in work practices could be beneficial to them as well. But we must begin by being honest and recognize that few of the skills appropriate within hospital buildings and centralized bureaucracies will be useful in a community mental health service. This will affect all workers from the consultants to the laundry workers. The main task will be to energize and enthuse workers and managers to adopt change.

In Manchester there are few examples of successful attempts to create new kinds of services. We would echo David Towell's view:

> So far in Britain there is no local project which demonstrates the complete relocation of hospital provision. All our contributors are in the position of still 'travelling hopefully' rather than having arrived.[3]

However, there are some signs that alternatives are emerging both within the health service and from the non-statutory sector in spite of the medically dominated plans being put forward by the regional and district health authorities. In North Manchester imaginative schemes have been developed to orientate services away from the ageing psychiatric hospital, including the development of a community-based mental health centre organized on multidisciplinary lines with a strong non-hierarchical team approach. This project is providing a local service and is encouraging participation in the management and design of the service by the community within which it is based.

In the voluntary sector there are a number of innovative mental health projects which have shown the viability of non-medical approaches as well as meeting ideas of need that the psychiatric services have largely ignored. These projects are worth particular attention. *42nd Street* is a mental health project for young people. It was established to give a more effective and immediate service to young people, working from a clear non-diagnostic and informal approach. The emphasis is on the individual's potential for change and the project has developed a consumer-based management committee. The workers operate within two democratic structures which allows for consumer criticisms and views to be embodied within the project. And 42nd Street is a striking example of a project that has successfully forged a new way of working with people with mental health problems, even though its funding base is insecure.

People not Psychiatry (PNP) is a self-help network which makes no distinctions between consumers and non-consumers. It acts as an effective pressure group, but also meets social and leisure needs. PNP has been in existence for a long time and its formal meetings – which encourage discussion on mental health issues (amongst other concerns) – only represent a small part of its work. PNP gives people status, encourages people to ask questions and raise anxieties about their treatment and to gain support from others. It operates on a very small budget, has no professional support and is non-hierarchical.

Commonplace was established by the Manchester MIND group in 1982. It too is a 'network' but it has a meeting place in the city centre. Commonplace opens during the evenings and at weekends, at times when other services tend to be unavailable. Commonplace deliberately makes no distinction between consumers and non-consumers. Decision making, conflict resolution and other issues are dealt with by the group. Commonplace seeks to combat isolation and loneliness and meet social needs. The following description comes from the Manchester MIND Annual report:

> We all need to interact socially. The problem is the venue, Commonplace could be analogized to visiting a friend at home. The setting is down to earth, not clinical. The room is about the same size as your friend's front room and the fact is that to some people it is their friend's front room ... For those who visit on the nights it is open, they are safe in the knowledge that someone is there, that the door is open ... The situation now is that the spirit of Commonplace continues seven nights a week. People meet at Commonplace and then go to each other's houses and continue the process there.[4]

Commonplace shows that with a minimal budget and without formal worker support, self-help networks can be sustained by consumers.

Unfortunately the valuable experience gained by these projects has been largely ignored by the mainstream services and there is little evidence that they have had an impact on the policy considerations of the health authorities. So the question remains, however, of how we can develop a campaign both within the psychiatric services and society as a whole to achieve change and what kind of changes should be promoted? We felt the most positive way we could end this chapter would be to list ways in which this campaign could begin. We have taken two main stances – the need to increase our confidence about establishing community-based responses in our everyday work and to counter the tendency to see mental illness as the problem of the individual.

This list is not exhaustive and is only a beginning; add ideas from your own experience – whether you are a worker or not:

- We can establish a network of progressive individuals or join an established network which shares common aims and problems in developing a community mental health service. We can use this network for our own support (we all need it) and to support others.
- We can become propagandists in our own right (just as *Psichiatria Democratica* have done in Italy). We can disseminate information for our own network and we can ask others to pass information on. To ensure involvement of other groups we can establish forums for discussion by encouraging traditionally separate groups to come together, for instance, tenants' associations and relatives' groups.
- We can begin to use a language which does not refer to discriminatory attitudes and values. Terms such as 'chronic schizophrenic', 'personality disordered' and even words like 'psychogeriatric' are at best unnecessary and at worst deeply offensive in the same way that we find racist and sexist language. We must avoid medicalizing people's experiences in this way and counter it by using the descriptions of experiences offered to us when people express their own distress.
- We can build alliances with groups of service consumers and help such groups to link up with one another and have a voice by helping them have access to facilities which aid their ability to organize, for example, rooms to meet, printing facilities etc., thereby encouraging the organization of consumers into pressure groups.
- We can support the emergence of participation by service consumers and voluntary sector groups in planning, organization and delivery of mental health services. At the same time we can refuse to collude with activities which exclude users, particularly the exclusive nature of professional networks which unjustifiably demand confidentiality in matters that deny the right of reply by users or their representatives. We must be persistent in our enquiries about why information is denied; for instance, doctors should be open about the side effects of drugs.
- We can bring issues to trade union meetings (for example, conscience clauses in employment contracts for those nurses who are unhappy about participation in electro-shock treatments) and raise awareness among trade unionists and other professional associations of the implications for workers in the development of decentralized services. The need to protect jobs must be recognized but so should the benefits of work amongst the community. Our view is that this would

enhance relationships between workers and the community which will lead to a better understanding of mental health services and more motivation to incorporate and protect it.

- We can try to extend the democratic control of planning procedures which have traditionally been the closed preserve of distanced planning professionals. At the same time we can make links with others in policy-making bodies who are prepared to take up issues. In particular where local authorities are embarking on 'localization policies' and developing neighbourhood-based services we must ensure mental health is on the agenda wherever possible (or advisable), persuade progressive local authorities to develop their own mental health policies and to use whatever leverage they have, for instance through representation on district health authorities, joint funding initiatives etc.

- We can strive to effect change with, not to, consumers of our services; for instance, we can share skills and enable users to develop their own potential and abilities to help others and themselves.

- We can challenge the medicalization of people's experiences by assisting them to stay in control of their own lives. We should offer support where it is needed most – in neighbourhoods, workplaces and people's own homes – and try to ensure the least disruption.

- Relatives and friends carry out 95 per cent of caring for people labelled as having mental health problems; because existing services only intervene if and when this support breaks down, it is ultimately exploitative of this major form of support. We must develop a better understanding of how we can work within these informal networks of social and economic support. It is our experience that there are many people in the community who are prepared to help – not from a motive of do-gooding, but because they have experienced hardship or tragedy themselves and have become empathic to distress in the wider community. We must find ways of developing this undercurrent of potential community support and making mental health an open debate.

- Finally we can argue for our health authority, or department, employer, etc. to develop a set of principles from which a more coherent policy can be established. Such principles should be based on our rights to human dignity and personal autonomy. The service should acknowledge and build on good practice, be open to change and be accountable to users, the wider community, and to those who work within it. *Change requires participation – get involved.*

References
1. Read, J. 'Fighting Mad', *Social Work Today*, 28 January 1985.
2. Ibid.
3. Towell, D. 'Managing Psychiatric Services in Transition', *The Health and Social Services Journal*, 25 October 1984.
4. Manchester MIND *Annual Report* 1984–5, c/o 178 Oxford Road, Manchester M13 9QQ.

Unpublished Papers by Manchester MIND: 'What a social worker can do to promote good practices in Community Mental Health'; 'What a psychiatric nurse can do to develop a community based Mental Health Service'; 'Describing the Ideal? – A Community Approach to Mental Health'.

22

Changing Professional Roles in the Italian Psychiatric System

PASQUALE DE NICOLA, ENRICA GIACOBBI, SANDRA ROGIALLI

The need for a change in professional roles began with the need to change daily routine during the dismantling and restructuring of mental hospitals. The psychiatric system was based on segregation which required rigid separation not only between patients and operators but also between the operators themselves.

Before work on de-institutionalization began, psychiatrists, psychologists, social workers, psychiatric nurses carried out their work within mental hospitals in isolation by following precise rules laid down in the handbook. For example, up until the end of the 1960s, psychiatric welfare in Arezzo was limited to containing disorders within walled buildings with the help of qualified psychiatric nurses, trained to this end, several heads of department, and a few psychiatrists including the director.

The only people with access to the department in addition to the nurses – who were segregated there with the patients – were the psychiatrists. It was they who processed requests from the outside and therefore had sole charge of any decisions. The social worker maintained contact with relatives and outside institutions in preparation for a patient's discharge when the psychiatrist considered it appropriate.

The role of psychologists, who were introduced as professionals into psychiatric hospitals and into the few mental hygiene centres set up after 1968, was essentially psychodiagnostic, intended to support psychiatric intervention. The 1968 law stipulated only one psychologist per mental hospital.

Nurses who were most in contact with patients and the department's daily routine were heavily conditioned in their work by rigid and circumscriptive regulations which denied them any community relationships. A high level of education was not necessary for nursing; in fact, many of them had only successfully completed their primary education. What was indispensable, however, was that they have a healthy and robust physical constitution and, if possible, a pleasant appearance.

The rigid hierarchy of doctor (head of department) vs. nurse–patient prevented any dialogue between its various components and created a situation where any new ideas, any creativity, were strongly suppressed; thus fostering an atmosphere of continuous anxiety. Nurses were required only to obey certain orders, often in written form, and if they failed to do so they were reprimanded verbally or in writing and admonished with fines or suspension. The patient had to play the role of patient and s/he was not allowed to complain otherwise s/he was confined to bed, or put into solitary confinement.

'Counting' and 'searching' were the main tasks carried out by nurses: the first to make certain that the patients assigned to them at the beginning of their shift were all present, the second to ensure that no patient was in possession of any sharp objects, blunt instruments, cords etc., with which s/he might damage him/herself or others; for this reason, nurses also had to check the number of items of cutlery after every meal.

Other tasks were ensuring that windows and doors were locked properly; administering drugs; distributing food; ensuring that patients bathed; accompanying patients to the hospital bar in single file with one or two nurses (according to the number of patients) at the front and at the end of the line; presiding over patients' conversations with their relatives (on Thursdays and Sundays) and referring those conversations to the head of department in order to ascertain whether they contained anything strange or dangerous; daily distribution of patients by therapy type, distribution of cigarettes or money owing; distributing food at mealtimes only to those patients whose families had brought extra; finally quietening down the numerous arguments between patients which could often arise just over the sharing of a dog-end.

Nurses were not allowed to socialize with the patients. They were often required to work continuous shifts with some overtime. Every day and every night was the same, one scuffle, one escape, more or less one suicide, someone who had to take the blame, no planning. This was the mental hospital where no-one except perhaps the doctor was able to have a therapeutic relationship with the patients.

The process of opening up Arezzo's mental hospital began in response to pressure from a group of nurses who, having been involved in the theory and practice of the Gorizia experiment, persuaded the administration to appoint Agostino Pirella – one of Franco Basaglia's most experienced colleagues – as director of the mental hospital. Some nurses and doctors were immediately opposed to the change; some, however, have since reviewed their position whilst others are still hostile. In effect the opening up of all mental hospitals questioned traditional psychiatry and the rigidity of professional roles, and highlighted the defensiveness of those who were hiding their own insecurity and personal deficiencies behind the status quo.

Making explicit the needs of very regressed patients forced all operators to respond to basic requirements (eating, dressing, acquiring a place for one's belongings) and to put aside their specific professional role. This process of acquiring new knowledge brought about restructuring and the continual questioning of previous roles in the search for new therapeutic strategies. Direct participation became the tool of work: patients, nurses, doctors, social workers, psychologists alike actively participated in morning reports, daily departmental meetings, chairing and minuting general meetings and various committees, for the purpose of examining problems and devising health plans together.

All of this facilitated the sharing of anxiety about death and destructiveness connected with mental illness, enabling people to do what one could on the basis of what was required at a given moment instead of 'somebody doing something according to a preordained role'. The doctor's central role became less important, allowing greater autonomy to those below him in the hierarchy. The worker who had the best relationship with the patient became the key therapist.

Consequently, the handbook became meaningless. This allowed the sufferer's needs and problems to be considered informally at various points during the day, and hence for the sharing of the medical-legal responsibilities. Outings to the town, trips and seaside holidays became possible as well as the opening of wards. In this way the residents no longer felt just imprisoned and controlled. Instead they each realized in their different ways that a part of society was interested in them and that they could be interested in society. Trust and hope were born again in them, which helped to put them on the road to a therapeutic programme and eventually to discharge.

This initial involvement, signalling liberation, was enough to achieve the first very significant results in the individual and collective rehabilitation of the residents and re-civilization. The first steps towards liberalization came when the workers and residents armed with sticks, pickaxes and spades demolished the high surrounding walls of the 'therapeutic community'; when the chronic ward was closed and transformed into a state school. The most regressed patients from that ward were transferred to other wards where, being in contact with less regressed patients, they soon managed to achieve astounding levels of rehabilitation. These levels were achieved by means of collective support, thus giving the lie to those who had thought that by placing a rotten apple next to a good one, both apples would rot.

The first home visits began by all workers, before and after discharge, and mental health centres were set up in the districts. Here a psychiatrist and a social worker, on a monthly basis at first, became the point of referral for the first discharged people who were receiving either a monthly benefit from the provincial administration or an invalidity pension.

Between 1974 and 1978 the above centres were consolidated and strengthened in five districts of the province. Psychiatric nurses, psychologists, psychiatrists, social workers and rehabilitation therapists joined the organizations and the real district work began, aimed at prevention, cure and rehabilitation.[1]

The workers found themselves immediately confronted with anxieties much greater than those expressed in the mental hospital; needs were more confused, 'defences' stronger and social support more difficult. The suggestion to set the group up as the therapeutic point of referral met with diffidence not only from the users but also from the health authorities and political/institutional figures.

Consequently, work proceeded slowly at first, amid many contradictions. Often the need emerged to identify the doctor as the most reassuring and powerful figure. The new style of working was cast in doubt by a highly structured social/health tradition and because the district service provided a diffused institution, whose mechanisms were more difficult to collate, explain and understand.

Despite these difficult beginnings, the experience we had acquired previously in the hospital allowed us to take our ability to understand institutional thinking and disadvantage outside, without having recourse to new segregational institutions (special wards, special institutions).

This type of teamwork allowed the individual worker to identify him/herself with the group plan and to acquire a sense of shared knowledge which helped him/her to feel confident when faced with the difficulties inherent in the work and above all with external agents (relatives, administrators, unions).

The leading role which this style of work emphasized placed everybody, worker and user, on the same level. It allowed each to identify with the other in that their purpose was to activate all the resources present for dealing with problems arising during daily routine.

Friendly, social celebrations organized inside the psychiatric hospital by both guests and operators were beginning, with the consent, active participation and economic contribution of the provincial administration of Arezzo. The parties had many purposes but the main one was to open the 'madhouse' to the people; they would then realize that 'mad' people were not the 'ugly, dangerous beasts' they had heard about (and whom many had never known) but that they were simply people needing a lot of social support.

The 'residents-guests' began to go out alone, not only out of the wards but out of the hospital; they began to walk in the town and go into bars and shops even though at first many needed the support of a worker; in short, they began to savour freedom and autonomy. The work did not stop here. It continued with actual discharges achieved by means of precise plans with the involvement and consent of the guests, their families, the operators and the neighbours; 'family groups' were created inside the hospital and the first collective district residence was tried, the post-treatment centre at Mugliano.

It is important to emphasize that nobody, whatever their ideas or politics, was claiming any longer that mental hospitals had a role to play or were able to provide treatment. Instead the discussion now was on how madness could be managed without mental hospitals. Although in certain instances initial hostility remained, the work carried out brought about a shift in and an enrichment of the debate.

At district level the teamwork of one group alone was not enough. Ordinary people needed to be involved and convinced in order to remove primarily the old idea of dangerousness which was rooted in the popular culture. Persuading and convincing people was the main task for the group members, every day, and in all circumstances where it was appropriate: in the family, in the general hospital, with politicians, with the forces of law and order, with general practitioners and in the street. All this took place mostly between 1978 and 1983 with good results.

For example, it was possible through close co-operation with teachers and classmates to keep at school a 14-year-old girl who manifested symptoms of 'schizophrenia with hebephrenic type defences'. By continuous integration over five years of the work conducted on the therapeutic side with the work on family relationships she was able to rely on her own abilities; continue to attend school; and take her examinations, once she had overcome the most critical phase of her illness. In this case, sharing the therapeutic project with teachers, friends, and school administrators as well as with the family, made it possible even with alternating phases to set the girl on the road to remission from symptoms and to an increase in personal and social autonomy. Both of these objectives have now been almost completely achieved.

The group of workers from the mental health service deals with mental health problems of all the district's population from birth onwards. There is close co-operation between workers dealing with children's problems and integration in the school and workers focusing on adolescents and integration in employment; and those working with adults.[2] This gives a unified overview of all the problems related to the mental health of a given population.

In addition, these workers contributed to the creation of other health and social services which had not previously existed in the district. For, once the structure of mental hospitals had been debated, the need arose for structures which had never existed in the district. Hence, the team already divided into various geographical areas was further subdivided into various services. This undoubtedly weakened its capacity to work according to the initial plan but it made possible a wider review and response to greater problems in the district. In fact, this work anticipated and gave rise to the 1980 general health reform law.

The latest legal proposals on health issues in Italy will bring about further changes in the organization of workers as the creation of a department of mental health is being suggested. With the Tuscan regional health plan (L.R.70/84), a department of mental health would be created which specifies within its structure a series of operative units and services organized according to profession. The following units are proposed: psychiatry (made up of nurses and psychiatrists), psychology; social welfare; recuperation and functional re-education; general medicine; medicine and basic paediatrics; and infant neuropsychiatry. All of these units co-ordinate in order to carry out the mental health plan.

This new organization has the advantage that it places emphasis on the concept of health rather than illness and sanctions the involvement of new functions and capacities, thus breaking the isolation in which psychiatry has been left for many years.

However, there are risks in this type of work organization. The physical division of workers means it will be more difficult to review a person's problems as part of everyday work. The potential clash with power politics and institutional engineering inherent in this organizational plan carries the risk of workers hiding themselves defensively behind sterile professional roles. The possibility therefore of corporate retrenchment in individual professions is greatly increased; a risk which is accentuated also by the increase in the number of intermediaries and in their level of power. In psychiatric hospitals, the director held maximum authority; at the present time, several authorities are being suggested who would hold differing positions. Such risks can only be contained by a well thought out professional/political programme. This must pull together all the knowledge, ability and power levels which have been acquired by experience, into a plan which, having set up the new organization along the above lines, will resume and accomplish the initial project, both outside and within the specific contribution which each individual professional figure can make. To achieve this, the point of departure must continue to be the needs and requirements of the most marginal and regressed in society for whom only a shared plan of work is effective.

At the present time, in Tuscany, even the political signs lead one to believe that perhaps it will be possible to continue the dialogue and the integration of the numerous roles within the district. This would revitalize the collective work which, in our opinion, is the only type which gives positive results.

Note on Training

Before 1980 psychiatric nurses in Italy were trained on internal courses in each psychiatric hospital. The most significant requirement for these courses was a robust physique. Since then training for psychiatric nursing has been replaced by training for generic professional nursing. The training course for professional nurses takes three years and is administered by the local health authority under a mandate.

Social workers are currently trained in a three year para-university course. At present, there are demands to make this a degree course of four years' duration.

Between 1971 and 1985, psychologists in Italy were trained in four year university courses; in 1985 these courses were restructured and lengthened to five years. Postgraduate specialist courses are also in the process of reorganization.

Psychiatrists are trained in medical school for six years. The practical component is not obligatory, however, and individual students have to make their own arrangements as to where and for how long it will be.

Concerning traineeship in general, new workers are involved in all stages of the therapy plan according to the individual user and/or service. At no time are trainees excluded, a priori, from clinical consultations to home visits and team meetings, unless there are specific reasons which are explained and discussed. At the present time, service workers are encouraged to participate in service training programmes for nurses.

References

1. Tranchina, P., Serra, P. (1982) 'Community Work and Participation in the New Italian Psychiatric Legislation', Stierlin, H., et al. (eds) *Psychological Intervention and Schizophrenia: An International View*, Springer Verlag, New York, pp. 109–20.

2. Martini, P. et al. (1985) 'A Model of a Single Comprehensive Mental Health Service for a Catchment Area: A Community Alternative to Hospitalisation', *Acta Psychiatrica Scandinavia*, no. 316, vol. 71, pp. 96–120.

23
The Case for the 'Re-professionalized' Psychiatrist in Britain

HAROLD BOURNE

Not long ago, in London, some astute medical students beseeched one of their teachers to explain why on earth they should give importance to psychiatry. After all, it only amounted to administering two kinds of pill – tranquillizers and anti-depressants – as they had come to understand for themselves when doing their stint in various psychiatric settings. Now, in fact, when professional utterances, official policies, and statements of virtuous intent concerning psychiatry in Britain are put aside, these medical students had merely discovered what, for clients, is a commonplace: they can expect pills, usually wrapped in sympathy, and seldom much else. Moreover, those who speak for orthodox psychiatry tend to be censorious of people who would have it otherwise. For there are psychiatrists for whom social issues and institutions, philosophies and political systems, the arts and creativity, form a central band in the spectrum of professional learning and theorizing.

This fixed irrelevance of psychiatry to human affairs and problems, in the ordinary meaning of those terms, is laid bare in public every time a psychiatrist appears in court. There, people who in any commonsense judgement behave in an abnormal fashion, and whose life has been a crippling sequence of childhood calamity and adult self-defeats, will be proclaimed by the psychiatrist as not suffering from mental illness. Or s/he will advise that it is a case of 'personality disorder' (a catch-all term for anyone who departs from average, especially if a misfit or social nuisance as well). Further it will be explained that no treatment is possible. Commonly enough, the psychiatrist senses a duty to neither so great as to keep 'his' hospital free of troublesome people.

Thus, he behaves unselfconsciously and unembarrassedly in this circumstance, as if deprivation, delinquency, ruined lives, and gross deviations of conduct were hardly any business of his. This abdication of responsibility has become habitual. The diagnosis of 'no mental illness' or of 'personality disorder' can absolve the psychiatrist from any therapeutic responsibility, if he so chooses, in cases of attempted suicide, drug addiction, sexual abnormality, marital difficulty, child abuse. This is so regardless of his wide range of studies and experience, and the incomparable medical heritage of clinical skills and lore which gives the doctor–patient relationship its singular qualities. Undeniably there is a role for other professions in the alleviation of suffering. But when the psychiatrist justifies this by saying they have skills which he has not needed to acquire, it is not modesty that activates him but a monumental incomprehension of what psychological disturbance (including 'mental illness') is about.

The irrelevance of this type of psychiatry to life, people, and their turmoils likewise seems to be on display sometimes in the clinical case conferences that are a regular psychiatric ritual. The 'case' is presented with an account of the symptoms and their onset, followed by a 'personal history' and a 'family history' in unassimilated detail (for example, a woman with doubtful epilepsy decades previously having no mention of a miscarriage three years ago). Nowhere to be heard is a word of her desires, disappointments, daydreams, of how she became what uniquely she is, of how she sees herself as a woman and a mother, of what strengths she can muster and what changes she wants to accomplish, as opposed to what treatment might be prescribed. Above all, this process cannot put it together, how to make her and her problems intelligible, and discover what it all means. Instead there is debate whether this be a depressive disorder, or schizophrenia, or a bit of both called schizoaffective psychosis, or perhaps just a personality disorder with some elaborate 'attention seeking'. It would also be on whether one drug or another is preferable, and whether her thyroid function should be tested, though no one for a moment imagines it will be remarkable.

A group of fellow patients could do better at making sense of this woman, and when occasionally brought together for the purpose by some rogue psychiatrist, they will pool their unprofessionalized and unspoilt native ability to understand others, and often make a dramatically better job of it.

Contrary to popular belief and fiction, in reality the British psychiatrist is a humdrum medical person, quite unlike the Hollywood stereotype. He (or she, just as often) is very much a journeyman doctor, employed in large hospitals, caught up in their workings and in official expectations of them. If s/he is involved at all in any steady, and far reaching sense, with individuals, it will be quite exceptional. During the years of his/her apprenticeship, s/he has no experience whatsoever either of being engaged for his/her services and paid by a client personally, or of working independently, unhoused in and unsheltered by an institution, in a one to one clinical relationship.

Consequently, and unbeknown to him/herself, the British psychiatrist's outlook and training are governed by the requirements of massive and impersonal public institutions. It is therefore not so surprising as it first seems that, although clients come and go from the outside world, British psychiatry proceeds with extraordinary irrelevance to the stuff of personal existence in the world at large. Nor is it surprising that its language is ever more dessicated (for example, an overdose or cut throat is 'deliberate self harm'; hysterical invalidism becomes 'illness behaviour'; addiction becomes 'substance abuse').

It is no more surprising also that its research often leans heavily towards physiology and pharmacology, and even when it does not, it tends to be inconsequential or otiose. An outstanding example, because of its prominence and respectability, is so-called 'life event' research: over the past two decades, it has been found that depression and madness may be preceded by 'life events', a pseudo-scientific term for misfortune, bereavement, or tragedy. Heart attacks, apoplexy, and death were all known by the ancients to follow bad news. Widowhood and retirement regularly touch off illness and terminal decline. Hence the flurry of discovery about adversity and mental breakdown proving to be somehow connected, is more illuminating about the state of psychiatry and its scientific research than about anything else.

Finally, it is not surprising that mainstream British psychiatry, irrelevant, hospitalized, and drug-bound as it is, remains obdurately unaffected by psychoanalysis. This contrasts with the spread of psychoanalytic language and ideas in the Western world and in every related discipline. The level of knowledge of psychoanalysis expected for professional qualifications in psychiatry were provided in 1985 in *The Times* through a journalistic article by a thrusting new London professor. In a virtual set of schoolboy howlers, psychoanalysis was depicted as some charade 'behind closed doors' for persuading wealthy or healthy people to remember childhood wishes for sexual intercourse with their parents. It is as if the thousands of books and journals that make up only the technical literature of psychoanalysis in the libraries, contained nothing for the psychiatrist at all. Meanwhile, in Britain, if a young psychiatrist with an interest in psychoanalysis, applies for a job up the ladder, he prudently keeps that eccentric interest close to his chest. At the same time, his peers will pass their specialist examinations having read no more about psychoanalysis and sometimes much less, than brighter student nurses on his ward.

And yet, dry and remote from life in its medical white coat, 'scientific' but irrelevant and sterilized as it can be seen to be generally in its actual practice, British psychiatry is not the construction of fools. As an edifice of hard-earned clinical information and knowledge of a certain kind, it commands respect. There are always to be found psychiatrists in Britain who have survived intellectually undamaged, who are not swimming cosily along in the mainstream, whose work is lively and free, imaginative and growth promoting. They are the inheritors of an alternative tradition in their discipline which, if squeezed to the margin, has never become extinct in British psychiatry.

In the 1830s a one-time professor of medicine in London, John Connolly, took charge of the new lunatic asylum at Hanwell. He had a vision which took him further still from academe – the treatment of insanity without forcible restraint. 'Non restraint' led to other far-fetched ideas – he wanted the inmates to have a regime of education, classes in singing and drawing, and trained attendants chosen for their understanding rather than muscle. The managers of the asylum were unconvinced and, in any case, were disinclined to waste money on fanciful schemes. Connolly soon ran into barriers and frustrations that are curiously familiar today in the Connolly Unit which, being a psychotherapeutic community in the NHS, bears his unorthodoxy as well as his name, and which is housed in the very same Hanwell Asylum – now called St Bernard's Hospital. Over the years, it too always has to contend with admiration for its idealistic principles, coupled with moves for its closure, or for the withdrawal of its staff, or for its transfer to derelict premises, and other such tribulations.

Some 35 years later, in 1876, Sir George Thane, a physician and pundit of the day, pronounced that Connolly was unscientific, sentimental and unfit for the detached and painstaking work of medical research. Thus the professional judgement of psychoanalysis in 1985 quoted before from *The Times* replicates previous pronouncements.

In retrospect now, it is clear that the great movement for 'moral treatment of the insane' – by decency, compassion, reason, and by personal example – in fact died out with John Connolly in the 1840s. It has been utterly forgotten for 100 years as British psychiatry passed into its Victorian darkness from which it has not even yet liberated its thinking. The blame for this has come to be laid on the Victorian builders of huge asylums. However, there was another large, if paradoxical, reason for the descent of night over psychiatry. This is to be found in the meteoric explosion of medical science and its technology which promised with certainty to solve the afflictions of the brain and hence the mind. In that perspective, the milk-and-water therapeutic possibilities of personal relationships, influence, and understanding, became smaller and smaller beer until solid and sensible medical men of science ignored them altogether.

And so from 'moral treatment' to the fairly complete disappearance of personal understanding in British psychiatry, we arrive at its patron saint and John Connolly's unappreciative son-in-law, Henry Maudsley. For him, the 'mind and all its products are a function of matter, an outcome of interacting and combined atomic forces not essentially different in kind from the effervescence that follows a chemical combination or the explosion of a fulminate',[1] and: 'It is not our business to explain psychologically the origin and nature of these depraved instincts ... they are facts of pathology like other phenomena of disease'.[2] Evidently, a psychiatrist had nothing left psychologically to understand and, if his textbook is any indication, Maudsley well and truly understood nothing. The older humanistic-personal tradition in psychiatry acquired a new life and dimension with the Freudian movement in the new century. Yet the medical-impersonal tradition, with its apotheosis in Maudsley and the great hospital in London named after him, has kept British psychiatry possessed to this day as a discipline without a soul.

The contrast between the early and late nineteenth century, between the optimism of 'moral treatment' and the medical bleakness of Henry Maudsley, is mirrored today by comparing psychiatry in its most conventional practice, in hospital, with its least conventional practice, in the psychotherapeutic community. In the therapeutic community, the *client* is not conferred with an illness, not put in a category with a Greek name, and not invited to undergo cure. Instead, he must undertake to change as a person. This implies acknowledging a need to be different, namely that for his own sake he cannot any longer go on as he is. The client contracts to work at altering his psychological make-up and the therapist contracts to provide expert assistance in this task; the treatment is therefore a collaborative enterprise. In ordinary hospital psychiatry, we continue to be in the world of Henry Maudsley, where the *patient* is in the grip of an illness which can be classified and named – with no other significant personal change required. The task of the clinician is to identify the illness and label it correctly, and to administer the right remedy; the task of the patient is to submit to examination, and to accept that remedy.

Table 23.1 The Main Traditions of British Psychiatry

	Humanistic-Personal Tradition	Medical-Impersonal Tradition
Ancestry	'Moral' treatment John Connolly Freud and others	Kraepelin Maudsley and others
Concern	the person and his uniqueness	handicaps, syndromes, diseases
Diagnostic Aim	to understand the meaning and purpose of symptoms and handicaps	to categorize, classify and correctly label symptoms, illnesses, and handicaps
Therapeutic Goal	the person to change, to readjust, and to develop	abnormal condition to remit
Clinical Contract	collaborative enterprise in which the clinician is the paid expert and the client is his co-worker in his own case. Both are responsible for the work of therapy	clinician decides on the treatment and administers it and is responsible for it; patient makes himself available for examination and receives the treatment, i.e. takes pills, follows instructions and directive advice
Focus	on exploring the person's interaction with others, and especially with the clinician – the latter being a paradigm for interaction between the client and persons in his family and social world	interaction between patient and clinician is incidental to the treatment and there is no exploration of it

Typical	psychoanalytic therapy
	individual psycho-
	  therapy
	group and family
	  therapies
	art, psychodrama and
	  creative therapies
	psychosurgery
	psychotherapeutic
	  community
		pharmacological treat-
		  ments
		electroshock (ECT)
		leucotomy and psycho-
		  surgery
		prescribed behavioural
		schedules
		reassurance, advice,
		  counsel

The present state of British psychiatry may now be put into perspective. It has two traditions, but it is overbalanced in allegiance to the medical-impersonal tradition and has almost lost touch with the humanistic-personal one. Consequently, it is characterized by its remarkable irrelevance to human affairs already described here. Far from being an expert in understanding people, the psychiatrist rarely has any systematic training in the psychotherapies, or any serious knowledge of psychoanalysis, or any real clinical familiarity with childhood and personality in the formative years – and commonly he feels no need for any of this. As for society at large, its trends and politics, its institutions and their problems, orthodox psychiatry has, beyond epidemiological data, nothing to offer or say. Therefore, in Britain, community psychiatry is, strictly speaking, a contradiction in terms and it is only consistent in that it is viewed with mistrust by many psychiatrists themselves.

Can psychiatry in Britain be made relevant? The difficulties to be faced in such an ambition require a detour. The rise of scientific medicine in the nineteenth century split off the body, as an object of rich and fascinating technical study, from the mind which could not be studied in any such way. This both created a fictional figure, the 'patient', with no individuality and no social network, and eliminated that network from normal medical awareness and study. From all this, not only have Maudsley's descendants and British psychiatry never recovered, but medical practice *in general* in Britain has been permanently debilitated and disoriented, despite belated and ashamed attempts to make it look like a science with a human face.

The question can be rephrased – can the mind be restored to medicine, and the psyche be put back into British psychiatry? The question can also be expanded because medicine, with its prestige and power, has stimulated the development of two other major professions in the mental health field: clinical psychology, and social work. Both are housed as well in the same large and hierarchical government structures of the welfare state, which do nothing to humanize their clinical outlook. Worse still in Britain, neither possesses even the minimal ameliorative opportunity that exists in psychiatry to get out into the open air and freedom to pursue their profession with and be answerable, one to one, to people who choose and pay.

Given these questions, there is much to encourage the view that whether a nation gets the government it deserves, in Britain it certainly gets the psychiatry it deserves. This is reinforced by the British preference for coolness and distance in social discourse and encounters, the emphasis on privacy and anonymity, the avoidance of physical contact and touching, and the undervaluation of intimacy.

Less obvious, if no more promising, are other peculiar features of the English mind, and of culture and society in Britain: the bias towards commonsense empiricism, and the aversion to global theories and philosophies. The medical-impersonal tradition of psychiatry, and the lifeless scientism of academic psychology are only too harmonious with the empirical bias in the national intellect. Thus their remarkably one-sided practice, their skewed and narrowed outlook, and their lack of extensive social horizons, can appear comfortably normal and be taken for granted. The British psychiatrist may faintly have heard by now of the Italian psychiatric reform: but to learn that essential to it was a political and social movement, *Psichiatria Democratica*, involves alien notions that he cannot grasp, and confirms his worst suspicions of their purpose.

When it comes to restoring the mind to psychiatry in Britain, to socializing and psychologizing its vision, and returning it to balance and its humanistic-personal tradition, there are educational issues to be faced that go well beyond professional training. Long before the future British psychiatrist takes off as a medical student, he can already be lame and lopsided through the handicap of a British education. Medical students mostly arrive at the age of 18–19 from the science stream in school, which in England means they will seldom know one idea of Plato, what the Renaissance was, or if the difference between the French and Russian Revolutions matters at all. They will have been selected at interview by middle-aged medical men, similarly educated, usually on the strength of marks in physics, chemistry, and biology, plus signs of some 'broader interests', frequent examples being sport or music. The future psychiatrist is now to be handicapped further by medical education itself, and its stunning and dehumanizing influence described before.

The training of the psychiatrist in Britain would be hard put to undo these constricting and disorienting effects of education from childhood to medical school in this country. Some remedial measures do suggest themselves – a period of personal psychoanalysis; placement as a fieldworker in social services; attachment to an educational psychologist visiting kindergartens and schools. The Royal College of Psychiatrists, which like other such bodies in the professional establishment here produces magnificently enlightened reports and policy statements, nevertheless ordains in this way. Entry for the specialist exam can require virtually no more clinical experience than some years' employment in a mental hospital, supplemented by limited attendance in child guidance clinics and institutions for the retarded. The requirements are notable for the gross omission of clinical work fully covering pregnancy, infancy, childhood, and adolescence, and the family, which are fundamental to shaping any adult with whom the psychiatrist presumes to deal. Further, the flagrant absence of systematic training and experience in psychotherapy with individuals, families, and groups, and a failure to insist on work experience in relevant non-medical settings, ensure the narrowness of the training. As it happens, the Royal College might not be averse to any of these but its hands are bound. The reality is that the mental hospitals and psychiatric departments throughout the National Health Service have to be medically staffed, young doctors must be found to do this, and, without the prospect of a specialist qualification and career, they will have no urge to oblige.

The so-called 'basic sciences' on which the Royal College does insist amount to a peculiarly unscientific demand for biochemical, physiological, anatomical, neurological, and behavioural book-learning, with little or no laboratory component. The 'basic sciences' confirm his respectability, still somewhat recent; perhaps they make his speciality feel genuinely a medical science.

In conclusion now, it must surely be conceded that to put psychiatry to rights in its shortcomings in everyday practice, let alone to renovate it as a discipline, would be a formidable enterprise indeed. And yet psychiatry really *should* be reconstructed – to make it relevant to human existence, to people young and old, their disturbances and difficulties, and to the problems of society. This is necessary if the psychiatrist is to become not only medically but psychoanalytically and sociologically valid, and to enable the mental health services to be responsive, lively, personal, and democratic in spirit. In Britain, not only are the peculiarities of national character, society, and the education system daunting; the self-satisfaction of the professional and academic bodies in medicine and psychiatry, and the absence of any overt wish for radical change as opposed to a grumbling sense among trainees, add to the list of obstacles on the way to reconstructing psychiatry.

Perhaps it is misguided, after all, to talk of reconstructing and re-professionalizing psychiatry – to think about and look for cures. Is not the answer to invite the psychiatrist into the therapeutic community of public dialogue and scrutiny, where there is no cure but a mirror to see himself as others see him, and a helping hand in the work of reconstructing what he sees? One more case for therapy – heal thyself!

References

1. Maudsley, H.C. (1883) *Body and Will*, Kegan Paul, London.
2. Maudsley, H.C. (1884) *Responsibility and Mental Disease*, Kegan Paul, London, p. 154.

24

Crisis and Identity: Extracts from the Theory of Franco Basaglia

SELECTED BY MARIA GRAZIA GIANNICHEDDA

Introduction

The following text includes two extracts from two articles by Franco Basaglia. The first, which is taken from a text written in 1969, includes: a theoretical exposition; a reference to the experiment at Gorizia; and the spread of practices to change psychiatry which led to the law of reform nearly ten years later.

The second was written in 1979 and is one of his last works. Law 180 is almost a year old and Franco Basaglia reflects on the 'happy but difficult time' when psychiatry 'lacked identity'.

The Identity of the Institution

In medicine, clinical diagnosis – i.e. the observation and precise definition of several factors emerging from a given situation – is the result of a relationship between doctor and patient. However, the nature of this relationship is ambiguous since it takes place between the doctor and an anatomical body which is simultaneously an object of investigation and the catalyst for a second point of contact. It is a relationship between an individual and an entity which has no choice but to be an object in the eyes of whoever examines him. But even in general medicine, this type of encounter requires a certain level of personal involvement from both doctor and patient: the first brings to the relationship his own overall way of life (and therefore the system of beliefs and values which make him part of his world) as well as professional expertise; and the second accepts being treated as an object by the doctor because the patient needs to have before him a respect which will enable him to bear and overcome the anxiety of being 'ill'. If we apply this reasoning specifically to the field of psychiatry, it is obvious that however much one tries to treat a person who has psychiatric problems just like any other kind of patient, an encounter with the body cannot take place as it does with the 'organic patient'. At what level must it therefore take place?

In institutional relationships (which are the dramatic, practical expression of traditional psychiatry) there are only two possibilities, both negative. Either the meeting does not take place at all, and the patient, who was already labelled when he was hospitalized, is simply caught up in the hospital. Or it takes place with a body which by means of the depersonalizing action is assumed to be ill in some way. At this point, the nature of the approach to be taken is decided upon.

But since no-one is able to draw up an etiology or pathogenesis of mental illness, references to the patient's body as 'pathological terrain' are rare and lack a truly scientific basis. This means that we have no solid basis on which to found our principles. And when we are confronted with a patient who presents a specific, scientific problem, all we have are a series of names (which correspond to a series of symptoms) designed to calm our anxiety in the face of a problem which we cannot resolve. Classification of psychiatric syndromes represents on the one hand a sign of our impotence and on the other our aggression towards an illness which we do not understand: it is indicative of the fact that psychiatrists find it impossible to admit that mental illness is an unresolved problem and that this truth must be covered up with a purely quantitative description of the symptoms. Because of professional scientific ignorance, psychiatric institutions in a sense are absolved from their function of ideological cover-up.

But if we examine the mechanisms which generally underlie the encounter between mental patient and psychiatry, we realize that we are dealing with a particular type of object-relationship. Both parties in the relationship do not leave their territory. Each of them only projects a part of himself upon the other, and this then gets fed back. The psychiatrist compensates for his powerlessness by attributing a label to this syndrome (the label is a means of defence when faced with the problem of a patient); and the patient accepts his own illness through the medical illusion (since this is the only justification the patient can perceive for having to be reduced to the status of an object). The psychiatrist's level of involvement relates only to the mechanisms which have set this encounter in motion. The distance which he creates and maintains between himself and his patient (and so in the type of object-relationship which he creates) is evidence that the doctor finds it impossible to break free from the depersonalizing process. To what extent do these mechanisms correlate with the illness and how can they be treated?

In practical terms the so-called therapeutic relationship inspires dynamics which – when examined thoroughly – have nothing to do with the 'illness'. Despite this they play a significant part. What I am specifically referring to here is the power relationship which is set up between the doctor and the patient. This is a relationship in which diagnosis of the illness is purely incidental, an opportunity for creating a power regression game which actually determines the way the illness develops. The psychiatrist is endowed with almost absolute 'institutional power' within the asylum structure; or with so-called 'therapeutic' power, 'sapiential' power, 'charismatic' power, or 'imaginary' power. He enjoys a position of privilege with regard to the patient which as such prevents the encounter being reciprocal; and therefore precludes any possibility of a relationship. As for the patient – because he is a mental patient in particular – the more he wishes to escape the reality of problems he cannot face, the more easily he will succumb to this type of object-relationship since it is the easy option. In fact, his relationship with the psychiatrist will endorse the fact that he has been depersonalized and relieved of all responsibility. But this type of relationship will enhance his level of regression and make it unchangeable.

The psychiatrist then uses a form of power which does nothing to facilitate his learning more about patients or their illnesses. Instead the doctor uses it to defend himself from them. Drawing up a list of the symptoms merely acts as a screen between the psychiatrist and the patient allowing the psychiatrist to distance himself from the patient and the problems of his illness. If we believe that illness is only the result of changes within a patient's psyche, and not of interpersonal relations as well, then the psychiatrist can be permitted to remain detached as if he were a spectator viewing a situation which is as unfortunate as it is inevitable.

Seen from a different point of view, the psychiatrist himself is part of the patient's real world. He is another person, a contact within a disturbed, broken set of interpersonal relationships, a part of the patient's world as much as his own body. The doctor then is closely involved, and part of the patient's real world. He cannot extricate himself except by deliberately withdrawing and refusing to be a part of this world.

This is why psychiatric diagnosis has become a value judgement. When faced with the impossible task of understanding or reasoning around a problem, there is no alternative but to unleash accumulated aggression on the individual who caused it and who cannot be understood. This means that the patient is isolated and put to one side by psychiatry in its effort to find an abstract definition of the illness, codification of its forms. Psychiatry need not fear either that any of its possible findings will be undermined by the patient who is ignored in this way.

If we now want to succeed in facing up to the patient and the reality of his disorder, we must put 'illness', i.e. its nosographic classification, to one side, even though we have been submerged by a mountain of illnesses, definitions and labels. We have never faced up to mental illness, only denied it. Instead of accepting defeat and recognizing our own impotence, we have rushed to hide our incapacity by denying the individual we cannot understand. This is why diagnosis becomes a value judgement in which all the psychiatrist's aggression is directed towards a patient whom he cannot understand; when in fact all that should be done is to recognize, like Jaspers, that he is incomprehensible. What should be the sensible honest acceptance of our own limitations is actually transformed and fanatically divided into what we do understand and what we do not understand. The anxiety caused by our inability to communicate and understand must be calmed quickly by a process of labelling. This denies value to the problem in question and takes it out of its context. It is precisely for this reason that the labelling process is so aggressive.

By distancing the patient from our world, we are uprooting him from his real world, and turning him into an object which is isolated from its life-history, from its environment and even from its own life. In fact he is simply reduced to the state of an object by our aggression. This is why patients who have been taken out of their social context – where they still maintain some alternative (however fragile) which keeps them, through ties, in contact with reality – are stripped of all human factors. They are reduced, at best, to the status of an object for contemplation: an interesting case!

However, what should be pointed out is that in this game of exclusion, the illness is purely incidental. This can be witnessed by the number of external factors which determine the patient's new role when he is hospitalized. The process is a confrontation between two different elements, where the value of one is taken for granted and the value of the other denied.

But the more difficult the situation, the more therapeutic should be the relationship and the greater the variety of relationships on offer to the patient. The original meaning of the word 'therapy' is dual: that of treatment, welfare and service, and that of cult and adoration. Ignoring the second meaning which is obviously linked to the witch-doctor image, the original meaning of the word was a concept of treatment linked to provision of a service, in which the patient forms part of a reciprocal relationship with whoever is helping him. Therapy would then be based on the reciprocal nature of the relationship between both parties. In current practice this reciprocity partially exists only in privileged therapeutic relationships (i.e. the individual relationship between therapist and client); whilst it is systematically withheld in institutional relationships.

In relationships of privilege a modicum of reciprocity does exist on a contractual level. This is when the patient has an illusion of the doctor's sapiental power. At this time the patient is actually playing a different power role, i.e. an economic one about which the doctor in turn has an illusion. Since this is a meeting between two powers rather than two people, the patient – in this so-called free relationship – does not lie passively within the doctor's power. In this case the lack of real therapy cannot be put down to the lack of a reciprocal relationship for they are both moving on the same plane.

But it is the nature of the territory where such a meeting takes place which is ambiguous, since it occurs between the role of doctor (promoted of course by the myth of his own sapiental power) and the patient's social role. It is this social role then that provides the patient with the only guarantee of control over his therapy. What he keeps also are the ties with his own environment, his own life-history and his own responsibilities – all of which will contribute to keeping him in touch with reality where it will be recognized that he still has a valuable role to play. This will last all the time his social value provides him with effective economic value. Once this expires his contractual power with the doctor will disappear and the patient will begin his real 'career' as a mental patient in a place where his social image no longer carries any weight or value. He will enter the world of the institutional relationship where the former reciprocity (even if very ambiguous) does not exist, and the lack of it is not disguised in any way.

Here, the only source of power is the doctor who is a symbol of the institution's unique authority. The patient is systematically excluded. His only alternative is to identify with the institution whose physical structures reflect that which he must become. What else can a patient do in this environment – which is completely acritical and aproblematical and where his only option is institutional life – but submit, yield to the doctor or the 'superior' and become colonized? In this situation, the doctor – whether or not he holds sapiential power inside the institution – is already the object of a cult as far as the patients are concerned; he enjoys pure power which is inversely proportionate to the space (both physical and psychological) allowed to patients. It is the patients themselves who build this power for him which then rebounds back on them – by means of a gradual process of regression – and helps to keep them bound to their condition as objects.

By making diagnoses and using various techniques, psychiatry plays a part in the power game of the ruling class which has already established who has to pay and how, in order to maintain its own equilibrium. Apparently technical sanctions provide absolutely no therapeutic benefit in these cases. They simply separate what is normal from what is not, using as a standard a concept which is neither elastic nor debatable but static and closely linked to the doctor's values and the values of the class which he represents.

At the beginning of our action to phase out institutions, that which could be seen as the emotional rejection of a sub-human condition has been revealed as the inevitable result of a specific sociopolitical aim – psychiatry being only one professional device.

Rejecting mental hospitals and scientific classification has given us the opportunity to identify – by creating a new institutional dimension – the close link between institutions and the social system of which they are an expression. It also means that we understand how all professional debates conceal a number of political implications which are in direct contrast to the professional aim; and which undermine and destroy any practical effectiveness. If the operation of a social system containing psychiatric asylums was based on excluding disturbed individuals from a certain class, then the operation of a social system with new psychiatric institutions aimed at maximum professional efficiency must be based on the therapeutic act itself – provided this is interpreted exclusively as a solution to social conflicts which cannot be resolved by changing those experiencing them.

This is why action to phase out traditional psychiatric hospital institutions has been transferred from the professional field (i.e. rejection of institutional anti-therapy) to the political field; and it is action to reject a type of therapy which, if kept within our socioeconomic system, will only be repressed and frustrated in any event.

The Challenge to the Lack of Identity

[From the preface to *Il Giardino dei Gelsi* edited by E. Venturini, Einaudi, Milan 1979.]

The practical breakdown of class marginalization, implicit in the very existence of psychiatric hospitals, has brought about a law in Italy prohibiting the construction of new psychiatric hospitals and making provisions for the gradual closure of those currently in use. The solution to this practical breakdown cannot be fudged by creating a new theory of interpretation or a new set of ideas but which nevertheless leaves the reality unchanged. What is happening here is the opposite to what has taken place in other countries. There the problem has apparently been tackled by decentralizing the services for controlling deviation to district level. It has not however made any impact on the thinking that goes behind everyday practice in psychiatric hospitals. The endurance of social marginalization, with its mystique of illness and treatment, can only promote a similar way of thinking at district level and in the new services. And the return to the psychiatric hospital and the thinking behind it will be subsequently strengthened. What inspired the new law on psychiatric welfare was a struggle to claim the right to individuality within a scientific field which was rigidly positivistic. This struggle aimed at demonstrating that what existed was not 'nature' and that if planned, 'nature' could be changed; just as what currently existed had already been 'produced'.

Even if it is the result of a struggle, the law can only be the rationalization of such a struggle. But it can also spread the rationale for a certain type of practice and turn this into collective knowledge. Even if it is the result of a struggle, the law can create a climate within which the pioneering achievements of a few become more widespread. It can also widen the debate, make it more consistent and create common bases for action. This is because this law sets out to achieve what has already often been foreseen, i.e. transfer of the struggle from a few people to an increasing number; even if this does mean slowly abandoning the practices of the first pioneering experiences.

In this sense the law has tried to change, or at least diminish the heroism, romanticism and perhaps the rhetoric which we were all suffering from. It has compelled us to confront what has been done in our time with greater rigour – this too is the result of our angry practice against the institution. This law has also exerted pressure in some way on the alternative psychiatric worker and has changed his/her consciousness of him/herself and his/her work. And now it is as if s/he were aware of the loss of that 'faith' which inspired us during the time leading up to the new law. Yet the characteristics of the newly emerging lay members have yet to be defined.

Today, after the passing of the law, we all find ourselves therefore in the atmosphere of quest and anticipation which characterizes every single course of treatment between what has been achieved and what still has to be done. The people interviewed in this book are aware of this situation and express the desire to fill this gap – a gap which indicates the lack of identity and historical perspective in our work.

Traditional psychiatry offered to the worker a precise identity as a guarantor of social control; just as the phasing out of psychiatric hospitals offered another identity – i.e. the rejection of this control. But now this rejection has been accomplished and the law confirming it has been implemented the need to progress further has emerged. Clearly the possibility of the liberating role – identifiable during the struggle against psychiatric hospitals – existing alongside any new role has diminished.

However, psychiatrists must continue to deal with individual suffering, though this still remains within a precise definition of the norm. These normal limits move, expand and contract according to need and changing social values. However, what must always be maintained is a clear definition of the limits. But the way in which suffering still expresses itself is rigid and confined within the classic parameters of mental illness. This is because the culture which determines people who are suffering from psychiatric problems (who feel they are on the brink, on the point of stepping over the normal limit, even though they know punishment and sanctions exist beyond it) remains the same.

Once the psychology of the psychiatric hospital has been broken – i.e. sanctions for the abnormal – psychiatric workers are at a loss when they meet patients who still move according to the old parameters of 'illness', and who hide and defend themselves behind these parameters. So identifying with the institution is no longer possible because psychiatric hospitals have been revealed as a form of defence for the sane against the sick; identifying with psychiatry is no longer possible because this has been revealed as the instrument which allowed the sane world to defend itself by creating a 'sick' place; and it is no longer possible to identify with the role of people who struggle against the psychiatric hospitals, because a law exists which has pronounced this institution dead. Nevertheless psychiatry must continue to deal with suffering. And it must face this without devices and without defences – if it is to come to grips with the world of poverty where suffering comes from, and if it is to put suffering back into the context it was separated from once it was defined as 'illness'.

It is this lack of identity which currently poses a challenge for what could be a different way of practising 'psychiatry'. And it is in this ideological and institutional void that we will be forced to approach mental disorder, outside the parameters and devices which until now have prevented us getting close to it.

Filling this void, this moment of suspension, indecision and uncertainty with other ideologies could prevent us reaching a new understanding, in addition to the cultural frameworks which imprison us. It would be easy to fill this emptiness with interpretational theories which have already been tried and which rationalize our uncertainty. Italy, which is behind on a cultural level compared to other countries, is now ready – and this is demonstrated by requests and needs for scientific and ideological reassurance – to accept psychoanalysis, behavioural science, relationship therapies etc. Elsewhere their acceptance has left intact both the process of social marginalization and the psychiatric hospital psychology which justifies it.

But the focal point which may break up the new Italian law is class marginalization. This has been accepted by psychiatric hospitals and by psychiatry but no new theories have been forthcoming which respond to the crisis that has been opened up. This is why we are able to see clearly the unfulfilled needs, and the practical frustrations, which aggravate psychiatric problems; and we are able to perceive the real powerlessness which causes illness, once we have to look behind what those symbols were designed to hide. This does not mean to say that mental suffering is rooted in material poverty only (which of course is significant both as a cause of the problem and for the type of response which it receives). There is also social poverty which compels us to express our needs in strange and tortuous ways, i.e. through 'illness', because we are denied a more immediate form of expression.

The need for a new 'science' and new 'theories' is part of what is inappropriately termed 'ideological void'. In reality this is the fortunate time when problems could start to be tackled in a different way. It is the time when we are obliged to really relate to anguish and suffering, because we have been deprived of all the devices designed to protect us from recognizing it. We can no longer automatically relegate it to the status of an object within the frameworks of 'illness'; and we can no longer use new codes of interpretation which would recreate the distance which existed before, between those who understand and those who do not, and between those who are suffering and those who are offering treatment. It is only in this type of direct contact, without the mediation of the 'illness' and its interpretation, that the individual nature of those with psychiatric problems can emerge: now that this individuality has finally broken free – from the objectivizing categories of positivistic psychiatry where the practical outcome was the psychiatric hospital – it can only flourish within a relationship which does not restrict it.

25

Towards Normalization: Polarization and Change in Britain

SHULAMIT RAMON

The point of departure for this chapter is to consider the likelihood of the British psychiatric system moving in the direction of de-institutionalization and normalization from its present state in which de-hospitalization is already taking place.

In contemplating such a shift, it is necessary to start by understanding where British psychiatry is now in relation to users with severe mental distress, and what are the options open to it.

De-hospitalization and its Aftermath

As outlined in the introduction, the number of in-patients continues to decrease, while the number of readmission episodes continues to increase. Taken together with the data that more than half of those hospitalized stay for not more than a month, the majority of the clientele of the psychiatric services lives by now outside the hospital for most of the time. In this sense, de-hospitalization has already taken place.

Two psychiatric hospitals have in fact completely closed during 1987, as compared to none between 1959 and 1986. These two closures have several components in common:

- The initiative for change came from the health management, and not from the professionals or the community.
- All patients were assessed individually and went through a short rehabilitation stage inside the hospital.
- No attempt was made to change the hospital regime, unlike the focus on such a change in the Italian examples (portrayed in Chapters 16, 18, 20 and 22.
- The sites were sold to commercial developers and the proceeds used to finance the change (again, in striking difference to the Italian closures, one of which is described in Chapter6).

261

Beyond these similarities, the outcomes of closure in these two examples could not have been more different: the first was closed by transferring all of the residents and staff to other psychiatric hospitals, apart from three nurses who opted to work in the community. The second hospital was closed by moving most of the residents to group homes and hostels in the neighbourhoods from which they came originally. The staff moved to work in local community mental health services, in the group homes and in generic services for the elderly.[1]

Many more closures of large hospitals are planned for the next decade, yet there is no scheme which does not include psychiatric hospitalization in the future. However, the indications concerning the quality of life of the majority of those previously hospitalized for long periods does not suggest that either de-institutionalization or normalization have taken place, as illustrated by Mangen (see Chapter 5), Kay and Clegg.[2]

De-institutionalization (defined in the preface as moving away from a strictly regimented and passive lifestyle) and normalization (defined as leading an ordinary, unmarginalized life) are objectively harder to achieve than de-hospitalization. In my view this is the case because they ask a lot more than de-hospitalization of providers, indirect users, informal carers and the general public. While it is clearer that a radical change in attitudes, structures and the division of power is being advocated by the protagonists of the normalization approach (see Chapters 3, 4, 5, 6, 7, 8, 9, 21 and 22 of this book for specific areas of such a change, in both the British and Italian contributions).

Professionals' Views and Conceptual Frameworks

The majority of British psychiatrists and nurses working inside the hospital do not believe that it is possible to achieve de-institutionalization with people who have been termed 'long-term patients' outside the hospital. Furthermore, they assert that it would have been more beneficial for this group to remain in hospital because of their assumed fragility and the assumed sheltering capacity of the hospital.[3]

The conceptual framework of these professionals has not changed: it focuses on the view of mental distress as a disease and attributes the incapacities of long-term users to that illness, rather than to other factors. Therefore, the main mode of treatment should continue to be medical. In the current move to de-hospitalization, this group feels threatened in terms of its power base, the definitions of the professional roles, and its lack of knowledge and skills for work outside the hospital.

The minority in these two professional groups, the majority of community psychiatric nurses, occupational therapists, psychologists and social workers in Britain, believe that most of the current residents in the psychiatric hospitals could lead a better life outside the hospital than in it, provided the right type of support is made available. This is related to approaching mental distress as reflecting on unresolved problems in psychosocial functioning, with or without an organic cause. Consequently, the preferred mode of intervention is not medical, but personal and social support, and the building up of a better working repertoire of problem-solving strategies.[4]

Most people in this group prefer to work in the community. However, in many cases they too lack the knowledge and skills required for normalization work, which is not an integral part of their training. The conceptual framework of de-institutionalization and normalization is one still in the making. It therefore does not offer for the time being a coherent and comprehensive model for practitioners who would like to try it out. Nevertheless, some beginnings do exist[5] which stress the need for knowledge on attitudinal and organizational change, along with the knowledge and the skills required for self-care and social interaction skills.

The recent critique of psychiatry in general comes primarily from sociology and history of medicine.[6] It focuses on issues such as the nature of the controlling aspect of psychiatry, the treatment of specific groups by the psy complex (for example, women, ethnic minorities) and the development of different disciplines in Britain. While it is sophisticated in terms of the issues raised and the level of analysis, most of it is too removed from the everyday reality of psychiatry, and especially the reality of the users, to be of much use to those interested in changing the psychiatric system.

The frustrations of the pro-normalization group are not less numerous than those of the anti-normalization group, including:

- Facing the consequences of cuts in local authorities' spending and manpower to resources for people with mental distress.
- The unending chaos of the social security system means that people who left the hospital are doomed to a degrading dependency on the staff, and do not get the chance for a right start to their life outside.
- The lack of co-ordination among the health authorities and social services departments which implies delays, changes in plans, and watered down compromises.
- The lack of support to those indirect users who are informal carers.
- The quiet – and not so quiet – sabotage of preparation for living outside the hospital by hospital staff.

- The patent lack of imaginative day activities.
- The indifference of local neighbourhoods in which ex-patients live.
- The crisis and relapses of some ex-patients.
- The fear that the government's attempts towards the privatization of public services would lead firstly to a poor public service for people with mental distress. Secondly the government encourages the development of a private, profit oriented, sector which is more difficult to supervise than the public sector. Thirdly, it may result in the exploitation of informal carers.

These are some of the 'nitty-gritty' issues which delineate the gap between what has changed in the British psychiatric service and related services, and what still needs to be changed in order to achieve a greater measure of de-marginalization of people who suffer from severe mental distress.

A Changing System?
The title of this collection, *Psychiatry in Transition*, has been vindicated by the British contributions to this book, as well as by other recent publications.[7] All of these texts attest that it is a system in which a growing number of its main actors, albeit still a minority, are permitting themselves to question and experiment on a scale unfamiliar in Britain since the 1950s. This impression is reinforced by some of the joint initiatives of health authorities and social services concerning de-hospitalization and the resettlement of long-stay residents and staff from the hospitals which are closing.

The experiments range from empowering in-patients to run their own ward councils, after a period of initiation by ex-users (Nottingham and Newcastle), through the creation of a mutual support system for users by users throughout a British county (Derbyshire) (see Chapter 19), turning users to local activists (Hammersmith, see Chapter 11 above), to a new national organization of direct users and allies (Survivors Speak Out, described in Chapter 1), whose first national conference got a warm reception in quality newspapers.

However, reading the main academic journals gives the impression that very little has changed since the 1960s. Not even one of the above mentioned initiatives has yet reached the pages of these influential journals. Readers interested in becoming informed about the transition processes of British psychiatry find that they need to read the more 'popular' professional journals rather than the more academic publications. Even among the less academic journals there is not one published by psychiatrists which provides basic information about the many small- and large-scale innovative projects currently taking place in Britain.

The Introduction of Community Mental Health Centres

While only very few community mental health centres (CMHCs) existed until 1985, 50 now operate, and this figure will soon be doubled.[8] Yet again the differences in what they offer are considerable: some work as out-patients clinics (i.e. by appointment only, offer primarily individual consultation and mainly medication), others offer drop-in facilities and group activities side by side with appointments, while still others work as resource centres, i.e. as facilitators of mutual support and flexicare activities (see Chapter 19).

So far, there are only a few centres which offer overnight refuge.

The Growth of Users' Organizations

A number of new direct users' groups have been formed, focusing on advocacy and policy issues. Some such groups work on specific issues, such as the relationships between ethnic minority clients and the psychiatric system. Several of them are quite effective in putting across the message of the validity of their perspective, which is fairly critical of the current psychiatric system and the approach to mental distress as a disease.[9] Their alternative system is briefly outlined in Chapter 1. Most of them act also as partial support networks for those active in the group.

At the same time, indirect users' organizations – such as the Schizophrenia Fellowship – have become more prominent too in the public eye, and able to command more support among politicians than direct users.[10] These organizations oppose hospital closures because of fear of lack of adequate services without such establishments, though they are in favour of sheltered workshops and group homes for some direct users. Recently they have joined forces with the Royal College of Psychiatrists to attempt to legislate a compulsory treatment order in the community for people discharged from the hospital who refuse to take the prescribed medication. All direct users' organizations strongly oppose this proposal.

The Significance of the Proposed Compulsory Treatment Order in the Community[11]

This attempt to amend the legislation to include power over discharged patients who live in the community is a major departure with the past, and needs to be understood as such. This is the first ever attempt to limit individuals' freedom not to take psychiatric medication when they have been evaluated as fit to be discharged from hospitalization. The proposed order would enable enforced hospitalization to prevent an expected deterioration, rather than when it ceases to be a hypothetical possibility, which is the criterion for hospitalization at present. Thus a fundamental change in the reasons for hospitalization and the degree of power of some professionals is at the core of the debate around the proposed amendment. For the first time in the history of the British mental health system psychiatrists have found themselves isolated and unsupported by any other professional group, as reflected in responses to the Mental Health Commission paper on this issue. And for the first time direct users, professional and voluntary organizations have joined in opposing the Royal College of Psychiatrists.

The proposal follows the logic of greater control given to the police and the state in a number of pieces of legislation passed during the last few years (for example, the Criminal Evidence Act, the legislation concerning industrial action and picketing). At the same time it goes against the doubts concerning professional decisions and their power not to disclose information to users (for example, see the 1987 Freedom of Information Act and the debate around it).

Beyond the issue of personal freedom vs. the right of society to limit this freedom, the suggested amendment reflects also on the growing gap between psychiatrists and their clients about a central issue of psychiatric intervention. Psychiatric medication is the most prevalent treatment to be used in the British system, yet the doubts concerning its efficacy for either severe or mild instances of mental distress are greater than ever before among users and the general public alike.[12] The amendment reads like an attempt to quell the doubts and the gap, rather than to look at the reasons for it and finding ways of discussing it openly.

The overt motivation for the Royal College and the National Schizophrenia Fellowship is the wish to prevent the worst effects of de-hospitalization, in which people become homeless and drift into prison.[13] This is inferred from the American experience, without attempting to analyse what this outcome is due to: mental distress; lack of sufficient support in financial and network terms; and being evicted years after leaving the hospital when their neglected neighbourhood is being renovated and sold off for large sums which benefit only the owners.

The Media's Response

The number of television and radio programmes on mental distress has risen sharply since 1985. Most of them are sympathetic to direct users, but even more to the relatives.[14] Moreover, the different types of media have been increasingly ready to provide a platform for the users in which to express their criticisms of the psychiatric services and the professionals who work there. In this, the media reflects on the middle classes' disenchantment with professional expertise in general.

At the same time, in every case of violence committed without a clear motive, schizophrenia or psychopathy are proposed as the cause behind it.[15]

Polarization and Change Factors

Thus the most striking impression of where the British psychiatric system is now, and the reactions to it, is one of polarization: polarization in thinking about it, in form and content of services, among the providers, among the direct and indirect users, among policy makers, and in the message expressed by the media.

Polarization reflects best the map of change-promoting and change-blocking factors, as well as the depth of being in transition, when inevitably conflicts, ambiguities, contradictions, doubts and new solutions come to the fore.

Looking at the charted map of change-promoting and change blocking factors (Table 25.1), it may seem surprising that the same factors appear under these two headings. However, given the polarization outlined above, these factors are at the core of the psychiatric system and within them have divisions which represent the different directions towards which British psychiatry is being pushed.

Shortage of space allows us to examine only two more factors, which I see as the most influential, namely the attitudes of professionals and the government's position.

Professional Attitudes

The importance of this factor cannot but be restated: one of the major lessons from the American, Dutch and Italian experiences of restructuring the psychiatric system,[16] and from the history of British psychiatry too,[17] is how much the possibility of a real change hinges on the attitudes of the professionals.

They are the backbone of any psychiatric system, and will continue to be so for the foreseeable future. Therefore their readiness to adopt de-hospitalization and normalization matters. It matters greatly if they are interested in patients moving out of the hospital, or are overtly and covertly sabotaging such a move. Their attitudes are also important in enabling the general public to support the change, and in the influence they carry with the policy makers.

Some of the anxieties and apprehensions of the professionals have

Table 25.1 Change-Promoting and Change-Blocking Factors towards Normalization Work in Relation to British Psychiatry

Change-Promoting Factors	Change-Blocking Factors
Attitudes of a minority in all professional groups, including health managers.	Attitudes of the majority of psychiatrists and nurses.
Innovative services established by the minority of professionals and voluntary non-professional sector.	Majority psychiatric practice is unrelated to normalization principles, or counter-productive to them.
The de-hospitalization process underway	Treating de-hospitalization as a 'decanting' exercise.
A strong and innovative voluntary, not for profit, sector.	The beginning of a private, for profit, sector.
The government's determination to restructure psychiatry.	The government's ambiguity about the content of a restructured psychiatry and its lack of commitment to a public psychiatric service.
Loss of naive belief in professionalism by the British middle classes.	Increase of the controlling function of professionals, including in psychiatry.
The emergence of users' groups on the public map, especially in the media.	The prominence of relatives' organizations in access to the media and MPs.
	The stigma of violence and mental distress.
Learning from innovative experience in Holland, Italy and the US.	Using the negative aspects of experiences of other countries to block change.

been outlined above in the section on professionals' views. An additional important factor is the greater measure of competition for power outside the hospital among the different professional groups which compose the British psychiatric complex.[18]

Yet most of the British restructuring plans implicitly assume that the goodwill, the knowledge and the skills are there ready for the move to a new psychiatric system. Since the planners are on the whole intelligent people, simple naivety can be ruled out. Following the more optimistic scenario, the gap between planners and practitioners is at the root of this lack of understanding, where putting resources into attitudinal change is viewed as 'inefficient' and 'wasteful'. The less optimistic speculation would be that the planners do not attempt a real restructuring of the psychiatric system beyond its physical relocation, and therefore do not need to change the attitudes of many professionals.

Nevertheless, within the different professional groups, including planners, it is possible to see today a generational gap in attitudes. The younger generation seems to be more ready to question past dogma and solutions and commit itself firmly to the normalization path. It is this group which would have to attempt to change the attitudes of the rest, or at least to isolate its main opponents from power positions, if normalization work is to have a real chance of taking off in the field of mental distress. They would need to learn the lessons from the Italians, but also from recent developments in the field of mental handicap in Britain, where de-institutionalization has indeed taken off.[19]

The Government's Position

The Conservative government in office in Britain since 1979 has put more pressure for change in psychiatry and more resources into some parts of the services than any other government since psychiatry became part of the NHS in 1948.

There is no doubt that its major motivation in doing so is to cut down on public expenditure in the long run, and that it is using de-hospitalization and de-institutionalization as ideological legitimation for this end. However, this is not to say that we are up against a wholly cynical ploy: the civil servants in the Ministry of Health are also genuinely interested in an improved psychiatric service and recognize that what is on offer presently is unsatisfactory in a number of ways, especially at the level of services outside the hospital.

Beyond this generalized understanding they too depend on professionals and users for the specific direction of improvement. In this quest for guidance, they tend to rely primarily on mainstream professionals, for the obvious reasons of belonging to the same establishment and their natural inclination not to endanger the status quo. Therefore they are more likely to be less informed by the more critical, innovative, pro-normalization, professional lobby.

This has been exemplified in the publication of guidelines by their advisory board, which produced a blueprint for the continuation of the status quo.[20] Yet by now even the British mainstream psychiatric establishment does not speak with one voice anymore, and the Ministry of Health has been naturally more ready to listen to those who are for de-hospitalization than to those who are against it. While this does not secure the commitment for normalization, it nevertheless leaves the door more open to it than it has been until now.

The government is currently expecting the Griffiths report on the possibilities of establishing 'community care authorities' which will be responsible for services to people with long-term mental distress, together with groups such as the elderly. At this stage it cannot be judged whether the report will help or hinder the quality of the service to these users. But commissioning it indicates that the government is aware of some of the stumbling blocks in providing a better service.

Yet the readiness of the government to allow private psychiatric hospitals to open in areas where public hospitals are closing down and its encouragement of private, for profit, accommodation for ex-patients demonstrate the internal contradictions in its position too.

Although greater interest in mental distress has been traditionally demonstrated by Labour politicians and Labour health ministers, this has not materialized in attempts to restructure psychiatry under successive Labour governments. Presently, Labour politicians find themselves in a quandary over de-institutionalization, because it implies the loss of jobs to many domestic, low-paid workers and could easily lead to the exploitation of informal carers. The pressure put by the current government to privatize the NHS, including elements of the psychiatric services, is an additional reason for the apprehension of Labour politicians. However, they have not come up with alternative proposals and have not attempted so far to push for the redeployment of the non-professional workforce.

This is an exciting and frustrating time for an involved observer of the British psychiatric system like myself. The inherent dilemmas have come to the fore and are more difficult to deny than in the past. This in itself does not secure a specific future direction of the British psychiatric system. Some partial conceptual and practical solutions too have come to the fore. These need to be much more thoroughly worked through than they are at present, to ensure that more openings will be available for de-institutionalization and normalization work.

References
1. Reid, H., Wiesman, A. (1986) *When the Talking has to Stop*, MIND, London.
2. Kay, A., Legg, C. (1985) *Discharged to the Community: A Review of Housing and Support in London for People Leaving Psychiatric Care*, City University, London.
3. See, for example, the introduction to Jones, K., Fowls, A.J. (1984) *Ideas on Institutions*, Routledge & Kegan Paul, London, and the exchange of letters by Weller, Pilgrim and Ramon in the *Bulletin of the British Psychological Society*, November–December 1985.
4. Watts, F., Bennett, D. (1983) *Theory and Practice of Rehabilitation*, Wiley, Chichester.
5. O'Brien, J. (1983) *Community Support Systems for People with Severe Mental Disabilities*, Background Planning Paper for the King's Fund Workshop, 'Planning Local Psychiatric Services'; Ramon, S. (1988) 'Skills for Normalisation Work', *Practice 2, 2*.
6. Miller, P., Rose, N. (1986) *The Power of Psychiatry*, Polity Press, Oxford. Bynum, W.F., Porter, R., Shepherd, M. (1986) *The Anatomy of Madness*, Tavistock, London.
7. Barker, I., Peck, E. (1987) *Power in Strange Places: User Involvement in Mental health Services, Good Practices in Mental Health Publications*, London; Brackx, A., Grimshaw, C. (1989) *Mental Health Care in Crisis*, Pluto Press, London (forthcoming).
8. Sayce, L. (1987) Overview of British CMHCs, Annual Conference 1987 of the National Unit for Psychiatric Research and Development, pp. 2–5.
9. See Barker and Peck, ref. 8, and: Camden Mental Health Consortium (1985) *Mental Health Priorities In Camden As We See Them: The Consumer Viewpoint*, London.
10. See the series of articles on schizophrenia and community care in *The Times*, December 1985, written by Ms M. Wallace, an active member of the Schizophrenia Fellowship.
11. Mental Health Act Commission (1986) 'Compulsory Treatment in the Community': a discussion paper; The Royal College of Psychiatrists (1987) *Community Treatment Orders*, June.
12. Gabe, J., Williams, P. (1986) *Tranquillisers: Social, Psychological and Clinical Perspectives*, Penguin, Harmondsworth. Golombok, S. et al. (1987) 'A follow-up study of patients treated for benzodiazepine dependence', *British Journal of Medical Psychology*, 60, 2, pp. 141–50.
13. Braun, R. et al. (1981) 'Overview: de-institutionalisation of psychiatric patients, a critical review of outcome studies', *American Journal of Psychiatry*, 138, pp. 736–49. Lamb, R., Grant, R.W. (1982) 'The mentally ill in an urban jail', *Archives of General Psychiatry*, 39, pp. 17–22.

14. For example, 20 programmes on mental distress were screened between September 1986 and January 1987 by Channel Four, who published a book to accompany the series: Brandon, D. (ed) *Mind's Eye*, Channel Four Publications.

15. The headline on the front page of the Independent of 20 August, 1987, read as follows: *Matricide as the Schizophrenic Crime*, on the day after one man killed fourteen people, including his mother, before shooting himself too in Hungerford, a market town in Berkshire.

16. Brown, P. (1985) *The Transfer of Care*, Routledge & Kegan Paul, London. Rose, S., Black, B. (1985) *Advocacy and Empowerment: Mental Health Care in the Community*, Routledge & Kegan Paul, London.

17. Ramon, S. (1985) *Psychiatry in Britain: Meaning and Policy*, Croom Helm, London, Chapters 3 and 6.

18. Rogers, A., Pilgrim, D. (1986) 'Mental Health Reform: Some Contrasts Between Britain and Italy', *Free Associations*, 6, pp. 65–79.

19. A good example of these developments is provided by the publication of the journal *Community Living* in April 1987. The journal is formally committed to normalization, gives a prominent place to life stories of residents of mental handicap hospitals who now lead an ordinary life, side by side with reviews of projects, services and the literature.

20. Dick, D. (1982) *The Components of a Comprehensive Psychiatric Service*, DHSS, Health Advisory Service, London.

26

Italian Psychiatric Reform as a Reflection of Society

FRANCA ONGARO BASAGLIA

[It is fitting to end this book with the contribution of Franca Ongaro Basaglia who, together with her late husband Franco Ongaro Basaglia, was a member of the group which pioneered the Italian psychiatric reform. Franca Basaglia, a renowned sociologist, is now an active member of the Italian Senate, taking the issue of psychiatric reform one step forward into the arena of public debate – the Editor].

Any discussion today – ten years after Law 180 was passed – concerning the Italian psychiatric system requires a clarification of the significance attached since the 1960s to the mental hospital and the various types of social deviation.

One characteristic of the Italian movement has been the focusing on the transformation of mental hospitals into places where the needs of patients are discovered instead of these patients being repressed and hidden by a culture which does not understand their disorder and regards it as incurable. Hospitals were transformed into places where a new way of dealing with psychic disorders could emerge which would tackle the practical and global nature of factors constituting the suffering they caused. The struggle therefore was aimed specifically at the mental institution and its inevitable violence and also at the scientific ideology which has become dogmatic and has reinforced the incomprehensible nature of the disorder, and hence the 'diversity' of the sufferer. The Italian movement proceeded subsequently in the direction of criticism of both institution and science in the belief that a change in mental hospital practice would produce new knowledge and understanding of psychic disorders.

Another characteristic was the recognition that the mental hospital did not only contain 'madness' but poverty and deprivation which when they became intolerable could manifest themselves as madness. Thus the mental hospitals revealed a class dimension. Psychiatric practice in them served to conceal social problems by means of technical treatment which implicitly disregarded them as such. It was not a case therefore of examining just technical treatment and an outmoded, anachronistic institution but also of considering the very function of traditional psychiatry (and the mental hospital) as a system for controlling deviant groups. The disorder often played a secondary role in such cases. By operating within the relationship between the dominant rationale of our culture (namely that of material production) and the material and psychological deprivation characteristic of psychiatric patients, scientific and political action was possible: action which was to demonstrate not only the backwardness of the institution but also its discriminatory social role, a role previously concealed by the alibi of protection and treatment. Knowledge of the link between a rationale which excluded anything different and segregated deprivation allowed the movement to reach the heart of the problem. It avoided simple recourse to new technical treatment, which even in a period of innovation would only have continued to confirm the role and function of the patient, the disorder, psychiatry and the institution as instruments of social discrimination.

The Italian situation was peculiar in having revealed the nucleus of the problem as political practice, and in having forged the link between professionals and politicians which then led to the reform in the legislation. Having been conceived at the height of the first experiment at Gorizia, this link was strengthened – after years of attack, accusations and confrontations with both politicians and wider public opinion – between 1967 and 1972. During that period the country was experiencing the struggles of the students' movement, the feminist movement and the trades unions which – alongside the classic themes of exploitation – opened the debate on health issues inside and outside the factory.[1] The result of this highly intelligent political operation which aimed to link normally separate sectors eliminated the risk of the movement simply being absorbed into existing political structures and in this way concealing the specific nature of the contradictions prevailing. It also eliminated the inherent risk in an isolated struggle by enlightened practitioners who, in trying to cope on several fronts with the problem of mental health and its archaic institutions, would have only been able to propose a new technique as a substitute for the old without altering the real function of the mental hospital and hence the logic of social deviation. Through the recognition of the political legitimacy of the movement in the psychiatric sector the possibility of widening the debate from mental hospital segregation to social deviation was created.

Reform was possible in Italy because practitioners who were questioning their own role of power and traditional frames of reference, forced all political groups to face up to the weight of practical experience which had been going on since the 1960s. They have been able to demonstrate that psychiatry too was governed ideologically by radically changing the nature of institutions. The break with traditional thinking and the gradual rehabilitation of patients had not just highlighted the outdated nature of the institution but had in fact revealed the ambiguity of scientific opinion which endorsed the need for segregation and the use of that opinion for concealing social problems which needed remedies other than treatment and therapy.[2]

General consensus on these topics and the accompanying social pressure in the 1970s produced the new law on psychiatric welfare which can be considered as the outcome of a cultural and political battle strong enough to involve the whole country. One only has to look at the frequency with which the problem was debated in those years in the media.

However, though the Mental Health Act of 1978 was the point of arrival of a 20-year-long struggle, it should also have been the point of departure for generalizing that experience and for a cultural change in attitude and behaviour towards all forms of social deviation. The conflict initiated by Law 180 is of a more profound nature than simply overcoming the crudeness and backward nature of a branch of medicine: it has put forward for debate the rationale behind segregation and also that which promotes specialist techniques in order to control marginal groups in society.

This is the focus around which the current debate is centred, an issue bound on the one hand by the radical nature of the Act and on the other by the change in the Italian political scene since the beginning of the 1980s.

The psychiatric reform attempted to alter not only services but also social relationships by providing encounters which did not exist elsewhere. It was hoped that new structures would emerge out of the recognition that needs are unequal and these structures would then aim to respond to those needs without the framework of traditional theories of interpretation, already compromised by endorsing this inequality. Although necessary, simply creating district services was not enough to achieve the cultural change envisaged by the Act. Structures which provided no space for expressing conflict, conceived purely as a negative element, would allow users very little margin for self-identification in the new services, for recognizing those services as their own, or for using them without creating new forms of dependence and dispossession. So long as health services are contained within the old way of thinking which concentrates mainly on the 'illness to be cured' and ignores the subjective and objective needs of the users, they can only continue to produce chronic illness, dependence and lead to reduction in a user's autonomy and responsibility.

In recent years it has become increasingly apparent that the uni-directionality of technical intervention is the primary cause of rendering illnesses chronic or of people wrongly assuming themselves to be ill. The most effective measures of prevention seem to be those which take into account the overall nature of the factors in question since this approach makes the sympton comprehensible.

The cultural frameworks at our disposal however are still only concerned with dividing up overall needs and in isolating whatever manifests itself as a symptom. One example of this are psychotherapists who are basically trained for private practice. When operating in the public sector they are confronted with a fundamental contradiction which is not easy to overcome. This type of training produces a profession which expounds a theory on the need for selection, for choosing some patients and excluding others. But the public sector cannot do this since it must take account of all problems which are presented to it, problems in which biological, psychological and social factors are tightly interlinked. Psychotherapists who find themselves faced with these realities have two options: either they 'offload' the most difficult cases, those which do not align with the psychotherapeutic setting, or, if they are willing (as is often the case) to take responsibility for the complexity of a patient's problems, they find themselves at odds with that same training.

We find ourselves therefore operating in a sphere where the culture which we have absorbed – despite ourselves – is of little use. The new culture can only be created by the public sector taking responsibility for the overall nature of various problems, documented in the contributions by other Italian authors to this book. If these problems are merely repressed they can result in various manifestations of illness and social deviation.

However, the number of social and cultural public settings which had been opened in the climate of the 1970s has gradually diminished. The thinking about fundamental problems has been hampered by the tendency to rationalize and reconstitute these issues and to redefine them as demagogic and unscientific. The result is that the law is only being applied in a restricted way which emphasizes only one aspect, namely the abolition of outdated mental institutions by incorporating psychiatry into medicine. Any attempt to go further than this and call into question the established social order is condemned as an idealistic fancy.

In fact a process of disaffection on the part of those government forces which had favoured the reform has taken place. The reform which had required some very radical changes has consequently been left drifting. This disaffection has been increasing gradually where inaction and lack of resources for implementing the reform have been causing problems and difficulties in terms of local political consensus.

It seems that at government level they have almost been waiting for conditions to emerge which will force amendments to the Act. These conditions include:

- The absence of a national general health plan and of standards of regulation and co-ordination on the part of the Ministry of Health.
- The freezing of personnel recruitment.
- The lack of specific financing to ensure the creation of alternative structures.
- The inactivity of both central and local authorities.
- The resistance of employees who are far from being automatically predisposed to radical change in their working practices.
- The difficulties arising out of the initial implementation of the Act in which psychiatry found itself playing its former role of 'last wheel on the wagon'.
- The restrictions placed on public meeting places, first because of terrorism and then because of the worsening economic crisis.

All of these led to patchy results in which everything is dependent on the goodwill of individual employees and administrators.

Considering the circumstances, much is still being achieved where working practices are in line with the Act.[3] Yet in other places the Act has been disregarded with impunity and clients have been left either in the former mental hospitals or in the limbo of out-patient services for which even the law makes provision.

On the part of many administrators and workers there is almost total incomprehension of the Act's significance which means it has either been disregarded or devalued in its implementation. Similarly the universities – and the type of professional training they offer – have remained largely outside the process of cultural change which the reform was designed to promote. Training bodies must bear some responsibility since they have continued to operate in a cultural atmosphere where the scientific debate implicit in the Act has been denied. Administrative and operational inertia, the universities' corporate protectionism and defence of their untouchable traditional scientific canons have both endorsed government inactivity which had a vested interest in creating the appropriate conditions for reopening the debate on the Act, and attempting to take a regressive step.

Because of this almost total absence of aid, public opinion began to conclude that the law was 'wrong', and it is due to this continued lack of aid now running into the tenth year that amendments to the Act are now being discussed.

It is true that other reforms passed in Italy in the 1970s have met with the same fate and for the same reasons. But the shameful neglect on the part of the relevant authorities, administrators and workers who have refused to assume the new professional and social responsibilities which the Act required has often led to intolerable burdens for the families of sick people, burdens which do not emanate from Law 180. This state of affairs has given rise to a justifiable reversal in public support away from a reform which has been only partially and irresponsibly implemented by simply closing the former mental hospitals.

It is evident that resistance to the cultural change envisaged by Law 180 is attributable to a number of complex factors which have little to do with the problems of mental health. These are:

- The dominant safeguarding of corporate and private interests.
- Indolence or incapacity to act.
- Persistence of the automatic link between illness and public order.
- A refusal to see not only the illness which had been hidden in our welfare institutions but also the deprivation turned out onto the streets.
- The unwillingness to face up to these problems and the difficulty of replacing a culture where problems are delegated to technicians and institutions, with one based on tolerance and solidarity (and therefore of personal and community involvement).

Yet another factor must be emphasized: creating services which focus on social welfare rather than on medicine conflicts with the power of medical culture which continues to affirm its resistance to breaking the mould of the medical and institutional model.

The lesson which can be learnt from the struggles of the 1960s and 1970s can be summarized by acknowledging that social treatment of biological and psychological issues is what conditions people's future. So action must be taken against prejudice and discrimination before accepting technical diversification.

At that time, the recognition of the weight of this conditioning even on natural factors had opened the debate on all processes of people's objectivization and marginalization which might affect natural diversity. The new individuals who emerged at the time (women, young people, old people, the mentally ill, the handicapped, homosexuals, prisoners) were the symbols which rejected objectivization and marginalization. Now they have become the source of social conflict which demands to be met and experienced as such, refusing to be refrozen into 'natural diversity' which in fact has served only to confirm their social inequality. New family rights, the divorce law, sexual equality laws, the right to an informed pregnancy, the creation of family advisory services, laws favouring youth employment, psychiatric and health reform and prison reform are – even in their incomplete and unimplemented state – the products of this conflict which even now is not being faced constructively. The conflict questions traditional cultural certainties, which were only possible when traditional scientific certainty was based on the total object of one's fellow man. Above all, this conflict demands the creation of new forms of social behaviour which take account of all individuals making up the community, who until recently were unrecognized as such.

It is of course difficult to live with these new women, young people, disabled people, mentally distressed people, old people or drug addicts. The presence of these new individuals and their demands which must be taken into account seems like an act of violence made against us: but it is one which we must take responsibility for when it becomes clear that the solution can no longer be the rejection of these problems according to traditional roles, separate places or by total delegation to professionals. Any solution which attempts to deny the conflict has limitations in that it becomes essentially a response to the needs of those who have to bear its burden (i.e. the relatives of the mentally ill, of drug addicts, of old people, of handicapped people). But for those in whom the conflict is expressed personally through sickness, deviation, old age, it is always a case of the 'final solution'.

If we do not strive towards equality, which is the foundation for reform, then the economic crisis will be used only to cancel out all attempts at change initiated in the past. We run the risk of wasting the individual potential which has led to the mature response at a critical time regarding dependency in institutions and to the fostering of people's greater autonomy and responsibility and hence to less spending on health.

Nevertheless the inertia accompanying the discussion on amendments to the psychiatric reform bill since July 1984 leads one to believe that the debate is still open even within the parties proposing substantial amendments to the law. Time therefore seems to be in our favour in the sense that even at this late stage and in spite of all the difficulties, district services are beginning to operate in a small way throughout the country even if they lack the necessary quality. In fact, the first stage of the enquiry conducted on behalf of the Ministry of Health in four sample regions indicates the viability of the psychiatric reform.[4]

The potential for change still exists, given the necessary willpower, if adequate funding were to be provided for training and strengthening these services, instead of wasting time discussing amendments to the law.

Alternative solutions – in fact, a return to mental hospitals only with different labels – are put forward in a very contradictory and paradoxical national climate. The diminishing of tension, planning and social struggle would seem to confirm that the auspicious 'modernity' must inevitably pass through the cultural and human impoverishment of our lives and our institutions. Yet the ability and wish of the people to organize themselves more and more autonomously into associations, co-operatives, and voluntary bodies shows how this new culture has produced a profound change which will not be easy to erase.

References

1. Melucci, A. (1981) 'Ten Hypotheses for the Analysis of New Movements', Pinto, D. (ed), *Contemporary Italian Sociology*, Cambridge University Press pp.173–94.
   Basaglia F. Ongaro (1978) *Una Voce*, Einaudi, Milan.
2. Basaglia, F. (1968) *L'Istituzione Negata*, Einaudi, Milan.
3. See Chapters 4, 8 and 12 of this book.
4. Censis, *Indagine sulla Attuzione della Riforma Psichiatrica*, 1982–85, Rome.

Select Reading List

Basaglia, F., 'Problems of Law and Psychiatry: The Italian Experience', *International Journal of Law and Psychiatry* 3, pp. 17–37, 1980.

——'Breaking the Circuit of Control', *Critical Psychiatry* (ed) D. Ingleby, Penguin, Harmondsworth, pp. 184–92, 1981a.

——'Crisis Intervention, Treatment and Rehabilitation', *Alternatives to Mental Hospitals*, MIND, pp. 23–6, 1981b.

Battaglia, J., 'The Expanding Role of the Nurse and the Contracting Role of the Hospital', *The International Journal of Social Psychiatry*, vol. 33, 2, 115–18, 1987.

Becker, T. 'Psychiatric Reform in Italy – How does it Work in Piedmont?' *British Journal of Psychiatry* 147, pp. 254–60, 1985.

Bellantuono, C., Reggi, V., Tognoni, G., Muscettola G., 'Comparison of Practice in Hospitals and Community Mental Health Centers', *Epidemiological Impact of Psychotropic Drugs* (eds) G. Tognoni, C. Bellantuono, M. Lader, Elsevier, Amsterdam, pp. 171–81, 1981.

Bennett, D.H., 'The Changing Pattern in Mental Health Care in Trieste', *Crisis Crisis Crisis* 1, pp. 42–8, 1980.

Bourne, H., 'Misunderstanding the Italian Experience', *British Journal of Psychiatry* 147, p. 452, 1985.

Brown, P., *The Transfer of Care*, Routledge & Kegan Paul, London, 1985.

Brown, S.P.W., 'Politics and Psychiatry: The Case of Italy', *Research Highlights in Social Work* 11; *Responding to Mental Illness* (ed) G. Horobin, Kogan Page, London, pp. 114–29, 1985.

Crepet, P., De Plato G., 'Psychiatry without Asylums: Origins and Prospects in Italy', *International Journal of Health Services* 13, pp. 119–29, 1983.

De Girolamo, G., 'Misunderstanding the Italian Experience', *British Journal of Psychiatry* 147, pp. 451–2, 1985.

De Plato, G., Minguzzi, G.F., 'A Short History of Psychiatric Renewal in Italy', *Psychiatry and Social Science* 1, pp. 71–7, 1981.

Freschi, M., 'The Italian Strategy to Community Care: An Historical Perspective', *International Journal of Therapeutic Communities* 7, 1986.

Hanvey, C., 'Italy and the rise of Democratic Psychiatry', *Community Care*, pp. 22–5, 25 October 1978.

Heptinstall, D., 'Psichiatria Democratica', *Community Care* 17–19, 1 March 1984.

Hicks, C., 'The Italian Experience', *Nursing Times* 16–18, 21 March 1984.

Jones, K., Poletti, A., 'The Mirage of a Reform', *New Society* 10–11, 4 October 1984.

——Poletti, A., 'Understanding the Italian Experience', *British Journal of Psychiatry* 146, pp. 341–7, 1985.

——Poletti, A., 'The "Italian Experience" Reconsidered', *British Journal of Psychiatry* 148, pp. 144–50, 1986.

Lovell, A.M., 'From Confinement to Community: The Radical Transformation of an Italian Mental Hosptial', *Mental Health Care and Social Policy* (ed) P. Brown, Routledge & Kegan Paul, London, pp. 375–86, 1985.

Lovell, A., Scheper-Hughes, N., *In and Out of Psychiatry: Selections from Franco Basaglia's Writings*, Columbia University Press, New York, 1987.

McCarthy, M., 'Italy Achieves an Ambition', *Health and Social Services Journal*, pp. 552–3, 1985a.

——'Psychiatric Care in Italy: Evidence and Assertion', *Hospital and Health Services Review* 11, pp. 278–80, 1985b.

Marinoni, A., Torre, E., Comelli, M. 'Evaluating Mental Health Services in Italy', *The Statistician* 34, pp. 231–5, 1985.

Massignan, R. 'Psychiatric Reform in the Veneto Region of Italy: the State after Five Years', *Acta Psychiatrica Scandinavica* 70, 36–43, 1984.

Mollica, R.F., 'The Unfinished Revolution in Italian Psychiatry: An International Perspective', *International Journal of Mental Health* 14, pp. 1–2, 1985.

Mosher, L.R., 'Italy's Revolutionary Mental Health Law: An Assessment', *American Journal of Psychiatry* 139, pp. 199–203, 1982.

——'Radical Deinstitutionalization: The Italian Experience', *International Journal of Mental Health* 11, pp. 129–36, 1983a.

——'Recent Developments in the Care, Treatment and Rehabilitation of the Chronic Mentally Ill in Italy', *Hospital and Community Psychiatry* 34, pp. 947–51, 1983b.

Perris, C., Kemali, D., 'Focus on the Italian Psychiatric Reform', *Acta Psychiatrica Scandinavica Supplementum* 316, 1985.

Pirella, A., 'The Implementation of the Italian Psychiatric Reform in a Large Conurbation', *The International Journal of Social Psychiatry*, vol. 33, 2, pp. 119–31, 1987.

Ramon, S., 'Psichiatria Democratica: A Case Study of an Italian Community Mental Health Service', *International Journal of Health Services* 13, pp. 307–24, 1983.

——'The Italian Experience', *Openmind* 6, pp. 12–13, December 1983/January 1984.

——'The Italian Psychiatric Reform', *Mental Health Care in the European Community* (ed) S.P. Mangen, Croom Helm, London, pp. 170–203, 1985a.

——'Understanding the Italian Experience', *British Journal of Psychiatry* 146, pp. 208–9, 1985b.

Renshaw, J., 'The Italian Debate', *Care in the Community* 7–9, 1986.

Simons, T., 'Psychiatric Reform in the Welfare State', *Psychiatry and Social Science* 1, pp. 227–40, 1981.

Smythies, J.R., 'On the Current State of Psychiatry in Northern Italy', *Bulletin of the Royal College of Psychiatrists* 9, pp. 177–8, 1985.

Tansella, M., 'Misunderstanding the Italian Experience', *British Journal of Psychiatry* 147, pp. 450–1, 1985.

——Bellantuono, C., 'Community Psychiatry and Primary Care in Italy', *Mental Illness in Primary Care Settings*, Tavistock, London, 1985.

Thiels, C., 'High-Dose Neuroleptics in Italy', *British Journal of Psychiatry* 145, p. 212, 1984.

Torre, E., 'Planning and Evaluation of Mental Health Services in Italy', *Psychiatry* (eds) P. Pichot, P. Berner, R. Wolf, K. Thau, Plenum, London, pp. 71–8, 1985a.

——Marinoni, A., 'Evaluating Community Mental Health Services in Italy after the Closing of Mental Hospitals', *American Journal of Social Psychiatry*, V, pp. 66–9, 1985.

——Marinoni, A., Allegri, G., 'Lomest Psychiatric Case Register: Old and New Long-Stay Patients', *Social Psychiatry* 17, pp. 125–31, 1982.

——Marinoni, A., Allegri, G., Bosso, A., Ebbli, D., Gorrini, M., 'Trends in Admissions Before and After an Act Abolishing Mental Hospitals: A Survey in Three Areas of Northern Italy', *Comprehensive Psychiatry* 23, pp. 227–32, 1982.

Tranchina, P., Archi, G., Ferrara, M., 'The New Legislation in Italian Psychiatry', *International Journal of Law and Psychiatry* 4, pp. 181–90, 1981.

——Serra, P., 'Community Work and Participation in the New Italian Psychiatric Legislation', *Psychosocial Intervention in Schizophrenia* (ed) H. Stierlin, L.C. Wynne, M. Wirsching, Springer, Berlin, pp. 109–20, 1983.

Vanistendael, C., 'Prevention of Admission and Continuity of Care', *Theoretical Medicine* 6, pp. 93–113, 1985.

Vislie, L., *Integration of Handicapped Children in Italy: A View from the Outside*, OCED, 1980.

Williams, P., Bellantuono, C., Fiorio, R., Tansella, M., 'Psychotropic Drug Use in Italy: National Trends and Regional Differences', *Psychological Medicine* 1986.

In preparing this reading list we have been helped by the availability of a much longer list prepared by Dr G. Girolamo and Dr G. Tamminello. You can write to them for the longer list at: Primo Servizio Psichiatrico, Cremona Sud-Est, Viale Concordia, 26100 Cremona, Italy.

Subject Index

Name Index

(people, places, hospitals, organizations and reports)